T0231681

Psychosocial Resource Variables in Cancer Studies: Conceptual and Measurement Issues

Psychosocial Resource Variables in Cancer Studies: Conceptual and Measurement Issues

Barbara Curbow, PhD
Mark R. Somerfield, PhD
Editors

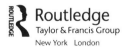

Routledge
Taylor & Francis Group
New York   London

First published by

The Haworth Medical Press, 10 Alice Street, Binghamton, NY 13904-1580 USA

The Haworth Medical Press is an imprint of the Haworth Press, Inc., 10 Alice Street, Binghamton, NY 13904-1580 USA.

This edition published 2013 by Routledge

Routledge
Taylor & Francis Group
711 Third Avenue
New York, NY 10017

Routledge
Taylor & Francis Group
2 Park Square, Milton Park
Abingdon, Oxon OX14 4RN

Routledge is an imprint of the Taylor & Francis Group, an informa business

Psychosocial Resource Variables in Cancer Studies: Conceptual and Measurement Issues has also been published as *Journal of Psychosocial Oncology*, Volume 13, Numbers 1/2 1995.

Library of Congress Cataloging-in-Publication Data

Psychosocial Resource variables in cancer studies : conceptual and measurement issues / Barbara Curbow, Mark R. Somerfield, editors.
     p. cm. -- (Journal of psychosocial oncology ; v. 13, no. 1/2)
     Includes bibliographical references and index.
     ISBN 1-56024-758-4 (alk. paper)
     1. Cancer--Psychological aspects. 2. Cancer--Social aspects. I. Curbow, Barbara. II. Somerfield, Mark R. III. Series.
     [DNLM: 1. Neoplasms--psychology. 2. Research. 3. Adaptation, Psychological. W1 JO858VC v. 13 no. 1/2 1995 / QZ 200 P97557 1995] RC262.P788 1995
616.99'4'-0019--dc20
DNLM/DLC
for Library of Congress
          95-23013
          CIP

ABOUT THE EDITORS

Barbara Curbow, PhD, is an Associate Professor of Social and Behavioral Sciences in the Department of Health Policy and Management at The Johns Hopkins University School of Hygiene and Public Health. She holds joint appointments in the Department of Psychology and the Department of Environmental Health Sciences at the same institution. Dr. Curbow received a BA in political science, an MA in educational psychology from the University of California at Santa Barbara, and a doctorate in social psychology from the University of California at Santa Cruz. Upon completing her graduate training, she was a NIMH-funded postdoctoral fellow in the Program in Social Ecology at the University of California at Irvine. She has been involved in psychosocial oncology research since the early 1980s and has published articles on a wide range of personal resource variables, including self-concept, self-esteem, coping, and optimism. Her current research interests include quality of life following medical treatment, treatment decision-making, the work-family intersection, and women's health. Dr. Curbow is on the editorial board of the *Journal of Psychosocial Oncology*.

Mark R. Somerfield, PhD, is a Research Associate on the Faculty of Social and Behavioral Sciences, Johns Hopkins University School of Hygiene and Public Health, and a member of the collaborating Faculty of the Center for Adolescent Health Promotion and Disease Prevention at the same institution. He received a BA in psychology from Millersville University of Pennsylvania, an MS in psychology from Villanova University, and a doctorate in public health psychology from The Johns Hopkins University. After completing his training, Dr. Somerfield was a Geropsychology Fellow at the Gerontology Research Center, National Institute on Aging, National Institutes of Health, and the American Psychological Association before returning to Johns Hopkins. He has been involved in psychosocial oncology research for approximately 10 years. His particular interests in this area include quality-of-life assessment, cancer and the self, coping with cancer, and research methodology in psychosocial oncology. Dr. Somerfield has published extensively on conceptual and methodological issues in research on coping with cancer, and he recently co-authored a chapter on personality and coping for *Handbook of Coping* edited by M. Zeidner and N. S. Endler.

Psychosocial Resource Variables in Cancer Studies: Conceptual and Measurement Issues

CONTENTS

Introduction

Barbara Curbow, PhD
Mark R. Somerfield, PhD

Much of the research in psychosocial oncology over the past two decades has attempted to document, understand, and explain individual differences in adaptation to cancer diagnosis and treatment. The impetus for this research has been clinical and empirical evidence that individuals with cancer, given similar levels of disease and toxicities of treatment, do not have similar levels of physical, psychological, and social responses. The importance of understanding the nature of these differences in outcomes is twofold: (1) early detection of people who are at risk for adverse outcomes beyond what would normally be expected might lead to more effective psychosocial interventions, and (2) an understanding of why some people with cancer are more adversely affected than others can provide insight into how people cope with serious life crises in general.

To date, the dominant approach in research on individual differ-

Dr. Curbow is an Associate Professor and Dr. Somerfield is a Research Associate, Faculty of Social and Behavioral Sciences, School of Hygiene and Public Health, The Johns Hopkins University, 624 N. Broadway, Baltimore, MD 21205-1996.

[Haworth co-indexing entry note]: "Introduction." Curbow, Barbara, and Mark R. Somerfield. Co-published simultaneously in the *Journal of Psychosocial Oncology* (The Haworth Medical Press, an imprint of The Haworth Press, Inc.) Vol. 13, No. 1/2, 1995, pp. 1-9; and: *Psychosocial Resource Variables in Cancer Studies: Conceptual and Measurement Issues* (ed: Barbara Curbow, and Mark R. Somerfield), The Haworth Medical Press, an imprint of The Haworth Press, Inc., 1995, pp. 1-9. *[Single or multiple copies of this article are available from The Haworth Document Delivery Service: 1-800-342-9678, 9:00 a.m. - 5:00 p.m. (EST)].*

ences in outcomes after cancer has been to assess the role of personal and social resources in adaptation. Although a variety of personal and social resources such as coping, perceived control, dispositional optimism, self-esteem, and social support have been investigated in the field of psychosocial oncology, little attention has been paid to the many conceptual and methodological issues surrounding the research. We developed this volume to provide investigators and clinicians with a systematic treatment of the state of the art in research on selected psychosocial resource factors. (We chose to limit the focus to personal and social resources, but we acknowledge the critical role of other types of resources, social class especially, in the stress process.) We also wanted to provide a careful consideration of more generic methodological and statistical issues in this research context. In this introduction, we review definitions of the term resource, discuss how the term has been used in conceptualizing adaptation to major life events such as cancer, provide an overview of some proposed mechanisms by which resources influence adaptation, and delineate lingering conceptual and methodological issues. We conclude with a summary of the articles in the volume.

A place to begin defining the term resource is with its common usage. The *American Heritage Dictionary* defines the term as (1) something that can be turned to for support or help, (2) an available supply that can be drawn upon when needed, and (3) an ability to deal with a situation effectively.

In the stress and coping tradition, Lazarus and Folkman (1984) defined resources as what a person "draws on in order to cope" (p. 158); resources are thought to influence individual coping processes. According to Lazarus and Folkman, resources can include both personal factors (e.g., health and energy, positive beliefs, problem-solving and social skills) and environmental factors (e.g., social support and material goods and services). Hobfoll (1989, p. 516) defined resources as "those objects, personal characteristics, conditions, or energies that are valued by the individual or that serve as a means for attainment of these objects, personal characteristics, conditions, or energies." Finally, Ensel and Lin (1991, p. 323) defined resources more simply and without reference to their function as "goods, both tangible and symbolic." They further distinguished between psychological resources, which are possessed by the person, and social resources, which are embedded in the person's social network.

In all these definitions, resources are represented as being inherently valuable; the definitions imply that resources facilitate attainment of some positive end state or avoidance of some negative end state. The definitions from the tradition of stress and coping in particular distinguish among various categories of resources and also imply that people have more or less of these resources. In summary, then, resources generally refer to aspects of the person or environment that are brought to bear on the maintenance or restoration of adaptation under taxing conditions.

There are two dominant perspectives on the role of psychosocial resources in stress adaptation research. One is the vulnerability perspective, which emphasizes the avoidance of stress-related illness (Holahan & Moos, 1991) and is rooted in disease models of human functioning and in models of immune functioning in particular. This is evident in Cohen and Edwards's notion (1989) that differences in social and personal characteristics "render some persons relatively *immune* to stress-induced illness and others relatively *susceptible* to the *pathogenic* effects of stress" (p. 236, italics added). In general and admittedly oversimplistic terms, the vulnerability perspective predicts that, under conditions of stress, people with low resources are at greater risk of experiencing adverse psychosocial consequences than are those with high resources. The latter are often said to be *protected* from these effects because they possess adequate buffering resources (see Rutter, 1987, for a consideration of conceptual nuances in this literature).

The second, and historically more recent, perspective is the resistance perspective (Holahan & Moos, 1991). The resistance perspective shifts the emphasis in stress research from vulnerabilities to strengths or adaptive processes. From this perspective, people are viewed more as active agents in the stress process and less as passive agents or "objects buffeted by external forces" (Thoits, 1994, p. 144). The active character of adaptation underscored by this perspective is integral to contemporary definitions of coping as constantly changing, conscious efforts to manage demands (Lazarus & Folkman, 1984). This active stance is also basic to compensatory models of adaptation (Thoits, 1994; Thompson et al., 1993). It is important to note, however, that the resistance perspective recognizes both ends of the health continuum, both pathology and health (Antonovsky, 1987). This is an expanded view of outcomes that allows room for consideration of more proactive adaptive efforts and positive outcomes of stressful life events (e.g., Curbow et al., 1993) but also preserves the notion of vulnerability, which is familiar to clinical oncology (e.g., Worden & Weisman, 1984) and arguably is necessary in light of the prevalence of psychiatric morbidity in this population.

A range of mechanisms has been proposed to explain how resources affect psychological and social outcomes. Because a comprehensive treatment of these mechanisms is beyond the scope of this introduction, we provide instead a brief overview of some general mechanisms that have been presented in the literature. (See Ensel & Lin, 1991, for a more complete review.) However, worth noting in the context of a discussion of general mechanisms is that the precise mechanisms by which resources affect outcomes are likely to differ for individual resource variables (see the articles in this volume and Curbow & Somerfield, 1991). This is consistent with Wheaton's (1985) hypothesized distinct routes of influence for specific resources.

Personal and social resources can affect adaptational outcomes through one or more of several different routes. For example, resources can prevent or lessen stressful appraisals: A potentially stressful event can be rendered either neutral or less threatening by the perception that sufficient resources (e.g., social support) exist for handling it (Cohen & Edwards, 1989). For someone who is already under stress, resources also may serve a preventive or ameliorative function to the extent that they eliminate or minimize the occurrence of secondary stressors that arise from the original, or primary, stressor (Pearlin, 1989). For example, adequate instrumental support (e.g., money, food) from one's social network can prevent or attenuate interpersonal stress linked to financial strains (Ensel & Lin, 1991).

Resources also may intervene between stress and its adverse psychosocial outcomes. This is the familiar "buffering" or protective function of personal and social resources. Further proposed in this context is that personal and social resources function primarily in the service of individual coping behavior. Thus, Gore (1985) distinguished between antecedent coping *resources* and event-specific coping *activity*: a coping resource (e.g., sense of personal control) is believed to exert its influence on adaptation through its effects on coping activity (e.g., initiation and persistence of coping efforts) (see Turner & Roszell, 1994). This is by far the predominant model of resource effects.

Finally, resources are believed not only to affect adaptation under high levels of stress but to have direct or main effects as well. As Wheaton (1985, p. 139) discussed, "It is possible to imagine support as capable of influence even when environmental stress is low—as in the continuing functions of a good marital relationship or the daily camaraderie of the workplace."

Empirical evidence supports this main-effects model. For example, social support has been shown to have salutary effects on mental health outcomes even under conditions of minimal stress (for citations, see Ensel & Lin, 1991). Holahan and Moos (1991) further found in a prospective community study, that three resources—self-confidence, easygoing disposition, and positive family support—related directly to psychological health. Notably, however, this relationship was observed only under low stressors; under high stressors, these resources related indirectly through individual coping efforts. Support for both direct and buffering mechanisms is available.

One often-discussed but surprisingly little-studied issue concerns the need for a match between resources and demands. Is it possible to have "too much of a good thing," as Wheaton (1985) proposed? This question has been considered most often in relation to optimism (e.g., Carver, Scheier, & Pozo, 1992) and perceived control (e.g., Wheaton, 1985), two personal characteristics that are generally believed to be adaptive. Whether those with generalized expectancies for good outcomes (optimism) or control (mastery) would tend to persist longer in ultimately futile and dispiriting efforts to change veridically unchangeable circumstances is an interesting question. Carver, Scheier, and Pozo (1992) pointed out that optimal psychological functioning requires people to disengage occasionally from pursuing a goal when continued effort is hopeless. Disengagement in these instances is adaptive in that one can work toward reaching alternative goals and life can move forward. These issues would seem to be especially relevant for studies of adaptation to cancer. As we have discussed elsewhere (Somerfield & Curbow, 1992), cancer and its treatment can block the fulfillment of highly valued life goals such as career advancement or child rearing. No one relinquishes cherished goals easily; people with high dispositional optimism or control may have even greater difficulty accommodating to such losses, although we are not aware of any empirical evidence that bears directly on this hypothesis.

Another issue that has special relevance for studies of the role of resource factors in adaptation to cancer concerns the cumulative effects of stress on people's resource reserves. Cancer is an intense, chronic stressor that over time might be expected to erode the resources of even the most hardy individual; those who go into the experience with less are at even greater risk of substantial depletion of resources (cf. Hobfoll & Lilly, 1993). The notion of resource erosion is helpful in thinking about the frequent observation in the psychosocial oncology literature that relapse is considerably more difficult to cope with than the initial diagnosis and treatment. Is this because one's resources have been depleted and therefore one has more difficulty marshalling the personal and social supports that are necessary to meet the challenge?

There are, of course, many other questions for research in this area. We can list only a few here. How do resources *combine* to influence adaptation? Are there core resources that are essential to adaptation? Can deficits in one area of resources be offset by surpluses in other areas? Do people reach a plateau where additional resources either are not helpful or are detrimental? How are resources related to each other? Do resources tend to *cluster* so that people are either resource poor or resource rich? Can people who have cancer be taught to develop, implement, or manage their personal and social resources in ways that will optimize adaptation? How can interventions be designed to permit accommodation to idiosyncratic resource profiles? How does the need for resources vary across the life-span? Do variations in the availability of resources occur across the life-span? Finally, what are the best strategies for measuring resources?

The first part of this volume contains five articles on what we consider to be core resource variables. Three of them focus on personal resources (perceived control, coping, and religion and spirituality); two focus on social resources (social support and family functioning). These resources were selected for review because they represent what many researchers consider to be the primary variables in the field or, as in the case of spirituality, a variable that is rapidly gaining acceptance. Thompson and Collins provide a cogent overview of the theories underlying perceived control, the most widely used measures, and further methodological issues. Parle and Maguire use the transactional model of coping to examine issues surrounding coping and the management of cancer demands. Jenkins and Pargament explore the role of religion and spirituality as resources in coping with cancer. Blanchard, Albrecht, Ruckdeschel, Grant, and Hemmick review the evidence on the role of social support in adaptation to cancer and survival of cancer. Finaly, Fobair and Zabora review the four major measures of family functioning. Following these five core articles, Spiegel offers an integrative commentary on the clinical usefulness of research on psychosocial resources.

The second part contains three articles that deal with important methodological issues in research on psychosocial resources. First, Gotay and Stern provide an extensive review and commentary on measures of psychological functioning that have been used most often in psychosocial oncology research. They provide a road map for exploring which outcomes resource variables might be used to predict. Second, Breckler provides a much-needed discussion of statistical and analytical issues in the use of resource variables. Finally, Waxler-Morrison, Doll, and Hislop discuss the roles of qualitative and quantitative approaches in exploring resource variables in psychosocial oncology research.

We hope that this volume is just the beginning of an ongoing discussion within the field of psychosocial oncology on the nature and use of resource variables. This discussion is crucial for several reasons. First, with or without structure and agreement, this literature will go forward. Researchers appear to be committed to using resource variables to explain outcomes. We believe that for this work to be truly meaningful and helpful, one must stop and reflect on what the work is producing. Second, interest in exploring medical outcomes–or quality of life–has exploded within all areas of research on adaptation after illness and medical treatment. That resource variables will be turned to routinely as explanatory concepts in quality-of-life research is just a matter of time (e.g., Brenner, Curbow, & Legro, in press). Third, there is the larger ethical issue that this knowledge should lead to tangible benefits for the populations it is intended to serve–namely, cancer patients. One growing concern is that, to date, research on resource factors generally has not translated into relevant clinical or educational interventions. Coping research, to take one example, has recently been criticized for failing to produce clinically useful findings (Costa, Somerfield, & McCrae, in press). Burish (1991) discussed this problem more generally with respect to anticipated calls from the public and from policy makers for concrete clinical dividends from psychosocial cancer research.

REFERENCES

Antonovsky, A. (1987). *Unraveling the mystery of health: How people manage stress and stay well.* San Francisco: Jossey-Bass.

Brenner, M. H., Curbow, B., & Legro, M. W. (In press). Proximal-distal continuum of multiple health outcome measures: The case of cataract surgery. *Medical Care.*

Burish, T. G. (1991). Behavioral and psychosocial cancer research: Building on the past, preparing for the future. *Cancer, 67*(Suppl.), 865-867.

Carver, C. S., Scheier, M. F., & Pozo, C. (1992). Conceptualizing the process of coping with health problems. In H. S. Friedman (Ed.), *Hostility, coping, and health* (pp. 155-165). Washington, DC: American Psychological Association.

Cohen, S., & Edwards, J. R. (1989). Personality characteristics as moderators of the relationship between stress and disorder. In R. W. J. Newfeld (Ed.), *Advances in the investigation of psychological stress* (pp. 235-283). New York: John Wiley & Sons.

Costa, P. T., Jr., Somerfield, M., & McCrae, R. R. (In press). Personality and coping: A reconceptualization. In M. Zeidner & N. S. Endler (Eds.), *Handbook of coping.* New York: John Wiley & Sons.

Curbow, B., & Somerfield, M. R. (1991). Use of the Rosenberg Self-Esteem Scale with adult cancer patients. *Journal of Psychosocial Oncology, 9*(2), 113-131.

Curbow, B., Somerfield, M. R., Baker, F., Wingard, J. W., & Legro, M. W. (1993). Personal changes, dispositional optimism, and psychological adjustment to bone marrow transplantation. *Journal of Behavioral Medicine, 16*, 423-443.

Ensel, W. M., & Lin, N. (1991). The life stress paradigm and psychological distress. *Journal of Health & Social Behavior, 32,* 321-341.

Gore, S. (1985). Social support and styles of coping with threat. In S. Cohen & S. L. Syme (Eds.), *Social support and health* (pp. 263-278). Orlando, FL: Academic Press.

Hobfoll, S. E. (1989). Conservation of resources: A new attempt at conceptualizing stress. *American Psychologist, 44,* 513-524.

Hobfoll, S. E., & Lilly, R. S. (1993). Resource conservation as a strategy for community psychology. *Journal of Community Psychology, 21,* 128-148.

Holahan, C. J., & Moos, R. H. (1991). Life stressors, personal and social resources, and depression. *Journal of Abnormal Psychology, 100,* 31-38.

Lazarus, R. S., & Folkman, S. (1984). *Stress, appraisal, and coping.* New York: Springer Publishing.

Pearlin, L. I. (1989). The sociological study of stress. *Journal of Health & Social Behavior, 30,* 241-256.

Rutter, M. (1987). Psychosocial resilience and protective mechanisms. *American Journal of Orthopsychiatry, 57,* 316-331.

Somerfield, M., & Curbow, B. (1992). Methodological issues and research strategies in the study of coping with cancer. *Social Science & Medicine, 34,* 1203-1216.

Thompson, S. C., Sobolew-Shubin, A., Galbraith, M. E., Schwankovsky, L., & Cruzen, D. (1993). Maintaining perceptions of control: Finding perceived control in low-control circumstances. *Journal of Personality & Social Psychology, 64,* 293-304.

Thoits, P. A. (1994). Stressors and problem-solving: The individual as social activist. *Journal of Health & Social Behavior, 35,* 143-159.

Turner, R. J., & Roszell, P. (1994). Psychosocial resources and the stress process. In W. R. Gotlib & I. H. Gotlib (Eds.), *Stress and mental health: Contemporary issues and prospects.* New York: Plenum Publishing.

Wheaton, B. (1985). Personal resources and mental health: Can there be too much of a good thing? *Research in Community & Mental Health, 5,* 139-184.

Worden, J. W., & Weisman, A. D. (1984). Preventive psychosocial intervention with newly diagnosed cancer patients. *General Hospital Psychiatry, 6,* 243-249.

Applications
of Perceived Control to Cancer:
An Overview of Theory and Measurement

Suzanne C. Thompson, PhD
Mary A. Collins, PhD

SUMMARY. A sense of personal control is associated with a variety of positive outcomes for those who are living with a chronic illness. The authors discuss the background and measurement of perceived control so that the construct can be used more easily in studies of coping with the experience of having cancer. They review four theoretical approaches that explain the role of perceived control and two current theoretical issues: (1) the situations in which control is and is not adaptive and (2) the origins of perceived control. The section on the measurement of perceptions of control reviews some widely used scales and discusses issues of current methodological importance: multidimensionality, primary versus secondary control, and central versus consequence-related control. Finally, the authors present a model for clinical applications of perceived control. *[Article copies are available from The Haworth Document Delivery Service: 1-800-342-9678.]*

Dr. Thompson is Associate Professor, Department of Psychology, Pomona College, and Adjunct Professor, The Claremont Graduate School, Claremont, CA. Dr. Collins is a Postdoctoral Fellow, Interdisciplinary Program for HIV/AIDS, Department of Psychiatry, University of California, Los Angeles. (Address correspondence to Dr. Thompson, Department of Psychology, Pomona College, 550 Harvard Avenue, Claremont, CA 91711-6358.)

[Haworth co-indexing entry note]: "Applications of Perceived Control to Cancer: An Overview of Theory and Measurement." Thompson, Suzanne C., and Mary A. Collins. Co-published simultaneously in the *Journal of Psychosocial Oncology* (The Haworth Medical Press, an imprint of The Haworth Press, Inc.) Vol. 13, No. 1/2, 1995, pp. 11-26; and: *Psychosocial Resource Variables in Cancer Studies: Conceptual and Measurement Issues* (ed: Barbara Curbow, and Mark R. Somerfield), The Haworth Medical Press, an imprint of The Haworth Press, Inc., 1995, pp. 11-26. *[Single or multiple copies of this article are available from The Haworth Document Delivery Service: 1-800-342-9678, 9:00 a.m. - 5:00 p.m. (EST)].*

An important part of human experience is the extent to which people feel able to obtain good outcomes and avoid undesirable situations as a result of their own efforts. This sense of perceived control, mastery, or self-efficacy is associated with a variety of positive effects, including better emotional well-being, enhanced coping with stress, better health outcomes, success at making desired behavioral changes, and improved performance on a variety of motor and intellectual tasks (Thompson & Spacapan, 1991). In addition, evidence indicates that feelings of helplessness and low control are associated with the onset of cancer and with faster progression of the tumor (Rodin, 1986). These varied effects speak to the usefulness of the construct of "perceived control" in understanding reactions to a traumatic situation such as the diagnosis of cancer. This article reviews theories about the effects of perceptions of control, discusses various measures of control, and presents ways in which the concept can be applied in clinical settings.

BACKGROUND

Research on perceptions of control has been stimulated by at least four conceptual paradigms that propose a central role for perceived control. An early approach, Rotter's social learning theory (1966), proposed that beliefs about the locus of influence on a particular outcome (internal to the person or external) and the value placed on that outcome combine to predict behavior related to obtaining the outcome. Rotter developed the Internal-External Locus of Control (I-E) scale to measure the first component of this approach—individuals' beliefs that outcomes depend either on their own actions or on circumstances outside of their control. The I-E scale has been widely used, and it helped draw attention to the concept of control.

A second influential approach to the area of perceived control is the theory of learned helplessness (Seligman, 1975). The original work in this area was based on laboratory experiments with dogs that exhibited helplessness after they were exposed to conditions with no contingency between their actions and outcomes. The learned helplessness paradigm was then presented as a model of depression in humans: people become depressed when they experience a lack of contingency between what they do and the outcomes they receive. Further refinements of this model added an attributional component stating that helplessness in the face of noncontingency will occur only if the failure is attributed to internal, stable, and global causes (Abramson, Garber, & Seligman, 1980). Thus, this theory assigns a key role in emotional well-being to feelings of a lack of control–the inability to obtain desired outcomes or avoid undesirable ones.

A third major approach that is related to perceived control is Bandura's cognitive social learning theory (1977), which focuses on one component of perceived control, self-efficacy–the belief that one has the ability to perform a desired action. Self-efficacy (i.e., "I can do this action"), combined with expectancy judgments (i.e., "I expect that this action will result in the desired outcome"), compose perceptions of control. Self-efficacy beliefs are most relevant to the area of making desired behavioral change because, in Bandura's model, action will be undertaken only when people believe that they have the necessary skills and abilities. This can become an important avenue for intervention to help increase behavioral change because individuals may underestimate their skills and need experiences that help them realize the abilities they possess. For example, Ewart et al. (1983) found that experience with a higher activity level and persuasive messages from medical personnel increased levels of self-efficacy in cardiac patients that led to higher activity levels in their daily lives.

Perceived control also is an important construct in social psychological theories of coping with traumatic life experiences (Janoff-Bulman & Frieze, 1983; Taylor, 1983). For example, Taylor's cognitive adaptation model (1983) proposes that adjustment to a traumatic event includes three themes: a search for meaning, reestablishment of perceived control or mastery, and the restoration of self-esteem. Traumatic life experiences can undermine a sense of control because the person was unable to exercise control and avoid a serious negative event. Added to this, control issues become particularly important as people attempt to terminate or escape from the stressor and deal with its consequences. Those who are able to maintain or restore a sense of control will cope better with the situation and experience less depression and anxiety (Affleck, Tennen, & Gershman, 1985; Taylor et al., 1991; Thompson et al., 1993).

These four perspectives illustrate the central role that perceptions of control are believed to play in the maintenance of emotional well-being, success at behavioral change, and the ability to deal with stressful life situations. The mechanisms that are responsible for the varied effects of perceived control are not well understood, however, and they probably differ, depending on which outcome is being considered. For example, according to the Mini-max Hypothesis, perceived control increases tolerance for pain and the ability to handle stress because it provides assurance that the maximum amount of suffering can be avoided (Miller, 1979). In contrast, self-efficacy may lead to successful behavioral change through a motivational mechanism–those who expect failure are not motivated to try making difficult changes in their behavior. Finally, perceived control may influence coping with a negative life event because feeling a sense of control changes the meaning associated with a traumatic event (Thompson, 1981).

CURRENT ISSUES IN THEORY AND RESEARCH

Research and theory in the area of perceived control has moved beyond establishing the effects of feelings of mastery and efficacy and is now focused on the complexity that is inherent in such a basic and multifaceted construct as "a sense of control." One issue that has long been of interest is the generalizability of the positive outcomes associated with perceived control: Is control beneficial for all types of people and in all circumstances? For example, theorists have suggested that, at times, people may be worse off if they believe that they have some way of exerting control in a situation, particularly if their efforts to exert control are unsuccessful (Burger, 1989; Thompson, Cheek, & Graham, 1988; Wortman & Brehm, 1975). This issue is still unresolved. Two studies have found that cancer patients are better off having a sense of control, even if beliefs in their abilities to control the cancer are disconfirmed by a relapse or progression of the disease (Taylor, 1983; Thompson et al., 1993). However, the participants in both studies were at early stages of cancer, so perhaps the disconfirmations of control were not strong or were unambiguous enough to have maladaptive effects.

Evidence that some people may be worse off when they are given control comes from a study of disabled or bereaved older adults who participated in an intervention study to enhance perceptions of control (Reich & Zautra, 1990). Adults who scored high in internal locus of control benefitted from the control-enhancing intervention, but adults who scored low in internal locus of control were actually better off if they were in the placebo contact condition that involved just social visits. Reich and Zautra (1991) suggested that those who are low in internal locus of control might prefer to rely on others rather than to enhance their own sense of control. Thus, perceptions of perceived control may interact with one's beliefs about the locus of influence to determine the effects of having a sense of control.

A second issue that needs attention concerns the origin of perceptions of control. Why do some individuals believe that they can control the course of their cancer and its effects on their lives, whereas others see little chance of having this type of influence? The severity of the disease and the nature of the objective circumstances one faces typically have only a weak relationship to feelings of control (Thompson, 1993), so other factors must be called on to explain the considerable variance in perceived control that is found among individuals who are facing similar events. Several possibilities have been raised. One is that orientations toward control are learned early in life, most likely from one's parents. In fact, Seligman and his colleagues found that the control-related attributional style of young adults is similar to their mother's style (Seligman et al., 1984). Other people may affect judgments of control in more immediate ways as well. For example, there is considerable evidence that the interactional style of family members and teachers can reduce feelings of control in young children, adolescents, and older or ill adults (Avorn & Langer, 1982; Boggiano & Katz, 1991; Eccles et al., 1991; Thompson & Sobolew-Shubin, 1993). Finally, the ability to find a sense of control in difficult circumstances may be related to one's life philosophy or more general orientations toward the world. For instance, cancer patients with pessimistic, catastrophic views tend to have lower perceptions of control, perhaps because they focus on the less hopeful aspects of their situation rather than on what could possibly be changed (Thompson et al., 1993).

MEASURES OF PSYCHOLOGICAL CONTROL

Locus of Control

Although two of the more well-known measures of global locus of control are presented here as a demonstration of generalized measures, these and other measures of global locus of control are not recommended. Instead, researchers are encouraged to use more specific measures of control (Lefcourt, 1991). One recommended and commonly used measure specific to health, the Multidimensional Health Locus of Control scale (MHLC) (Wallston, Wallston, & DeVellis, 1978), also is reviewed.

Internal-External Locus of Control scale. In the most widely known measure of locus of control for adults, Rotter's I-E scale (1966), locus of control refers to a unidimensional continuum concerning the causal relationship between actions and outcomes with internality (the belief that actions are causally connected to outcomes) at one end and externality (the belief that actions and outcomes are independent of one another) at the other.

The I-E scale is a self-administered paper-and-pencil measure that consists of 23 forced-choice question pairs and six filler items. For each pair of items, one response choice is external and the other is internal.

Although the I-E scale is widely used, it has measurement problems ranging from questionable discriminant validity to factor analyses that indicate there are two or more factors underlying the construct of locus of control (e.g., Collins, 1974; Mirels, 1970). Furthermore, the relatively low correlation between the internal and external locus of control items indicates that the response choices for each of the 23 pairs of items are not truly opposite or mutually exclusive choices. That is, a person could endorse both responses for each of the 23 pairs. Because of these measurement problems and the availability of more refined instruments, use of this more general measure of locus of control is not recommended (Lefcourt, 1991).

Adult Nowicki-Strickland Internal-External Control Scale. The Adult Nowicki-Strickland Internal-External Control Scale (ANSIE)

(Nowicki & Duke, 1983) assesses internal-external locus of control as defined by Rotter (1966). The measure was derived from the Children's Nowicki-Strickland Internal-External Control Scale and consists of 40 self-administered items with a yes-no response format.

The ANSIE has acceptable reliability and appears to have an underlying general factor of "helplessness," which accounts for 30 percent of the variance (Nowicki & Duke, 1983). The measure has acceptable convergent validity and discriminant validity.

This measure is useful as an exploratory tool to assess developmental changes in locus of control but is not useful as a predictor of psychological adjustment. That is, like the I-E Scale, the ANSIE is not recommended in research settings that require predictive validity (Lefcourt, 1991).

Multidimensional Health Locus of Control scale. The MHLC consists of 18 self-administered items measured on a six-point Likert-type scale. The measure has three subscales–Internal Health Locus of Control, Chance Health Locus of Control, and Powerful Others Externality–with six items per subscale. The internal consistency of the three subscales is low to acceptable, with good test-retest reliabilities within a test interval of four to six months. Convergent validity has been established with a variety of medical samples and is too extensive to summarize in a review article (see Wallston & Wallston, 1981, for a complete analysis of convergent validity). For discriminant validity, the MHLC is not significantly correlated with measures of social desirability.

The MHLC is a generalized measure of health-related control beliefs. Lefcourt (1991) recommended that disease-specific perceived control also should be assessed because perceptions of one's own control in a particular situation may be more important to adjustment than generalized expectations of control in health settings. That is, patients may, in general, have a high expectation of internal control over their health but may feel that they have no actual control over the effectiveness of their chemotherapy.

Measures of Perceived Control

In contrast to measures of locus of control, measures of perceived control provide more accurate predictions of psychological adjustment and, in some instances, future health status. As a rule of thumb, the more problem-specific the measure, the better its predictive validity regarding psychological and health outcomes. The following is an overview of measures of perceived control that are available.

Marshall's Multidimensional Health-Related Control and Efficacy Scale. Marshall's Multidimensional Health-Related Control Efficacy Scale (Marshall, 1991) consists of 14 items that are rated on six-point scales and is intended to assess the respondent's perceived control over and mastery of his or her health. The scale is composed of four health-related dimensions of control: (1) Prevention of Illness, (2) Management of Illness, (3) Illness-Related Self-Efficacy, and (4) Illness-Related Self-Blame. For criterion validity, the first two dimensions have been found to be correlated with health-related locus of control measures, and the Illness-Related Self-Efficacy dimension is related to measures of adjustment (Marshall, 1991).

The Prevention of Illness subscale assesses the belief that one can or cannot control the onset of illness. The Management of Illness subscale refers to beliefs that illness can or cannot be managed. The Illness-Related Self-Efficacy subscale focuses on the belief that one does or does not have access to the means to manage illness. This subscale was correlated with measures of adjustment to illness. The Illness-Related Self-Blame subscale measures the degree of self-blame for negative health-related outcomes.

Mastery Scale. Pearlin and Schooler's Mastery Scale (1978) consists of seven items that are intended to assess global beliefs of perceived control or beliefs regarding one's ability to control an event versus being controlled by fate. The scale is often used with medical populations to predict psychological adjustment.

Scale development. Because few scales exist in the literature for specific populations or situations, most researchers write their own measures of perceived control. This allows the researcher to assess the various components of perceived control for a specific medical population or situation. One strategy is to identify goals that are relevant to the situation, such as emotional well-being, obtaining adequate information, maintaining good relationships with family and friends, minimizing symptoms and physical discomfort, and preventing a recurrence. For each area, respondents are asked to rate the extent to which they can obtain these outcomes through their own effort on a scale ranging from "Not at all" to "A great deal." Of course, care must be taken when developing a measure to avoid the problems that can seriously compromise the reliability or validity of the scale. A thorough discussion of these measurement issues is beyond the scope of this article (see Anastasi, 1976, and Bailey, 1993, for psychometric issues in developing a scale).

In conclusion, researchers are encouraged to specify components of perceived control in which they are interested and to select measures intended for their specific medical population, medical situation, or both. Because there are many more populations and situations than developed measures of control in the literature, researchers will probably have to develop their own scales in many cases.

ADDITIONAL METHODOLOGICAL ISSUES

To date, psychological control has received a tremendous amount of attention, but most of the research asks the question, "Does psychological control affect adjustment to chronic illness and other traumatic life events?" This question is important, but what is needed now is a thorough understanding of the concept of psychological control and its many components. In this section, we discuss the various dimensions or components of control that make up this rather broad concept and the implications of this complexity for measurement.

Multidimensionality

Research with Rotter's I-E scale provided the first important glimpse of the complexity of psychological control. Factor analytic studies indicated that instead of being unidimensional, the scale assesses at least four distinct components or control beliefs: a world that is difficult versus easy, just versus unjust, predictable versus unpredictable, and politically responsive versus politically unresponsive (Collins, 1974). A person can be internal in some of these domains and external in the others. This fact led to the recognition of the need to assess control beliefs in specific areas of life rather than assess one's overall internality or externality.

Beliefs about perceived control can differ across life domains, and these beliefs can change as a person's life circumstances change (see, for example, Reich & Zautra, 1991). For instance, a manager can feel in control at work but out of control when dealing with her teenage daughter. Similarly, a cancer patient can feel in control of his finances but feel little control over the progression of the cancer. In addition, as adults age they tend to remain constant in locus of control, but their perceived control or ability to affect specific situations may change (Rodin, 1987), especially beliefs in control over cognitive functioning and health (Lachman, 1991). A distinction between global and specific control is important because the more specific measures, assuming they are well designed, are the better predictors of psychological adjustment.

Primary and Secondary Control Processes

Rothbaum, Weisz, and Snyder (1982) made an important distinction in two forms of beliefs about perceived control–primary and secondary control processes. Primary control processes consist of believing one's actions can have a direct impact on the situation. For instance, a cancer patient might believe that he can control a recurrence of the disease by changing his diet. Another cancer patient might believe that exercising more will speed her recovery.

Secondary control processes involve accepting one's lack of control in the situation. They include turning to others for help (vicarious control), believing in fate or luck (illusory control), reinterpreting the event to make it more acceptable (interpretive control), or attempting to predict events so that they will be easier to accept when and if they occur (predictive control). For example, a cancer patient may believe that she cannot control her cancer but her oncologist can (vicarious control). She might turn to her oncologist and passively follow his or her instructions rather than search for information about cancer and initiate interventions on her own. Another patient may believe that fate rules his life and that he can do little about his cancer beyond accepting the illness as his "lot in life" (illusory control). Still another patient might report that his cancer was, in a sense, the best thing that could have happened because it made him realize how fragile life is and the importance of being with family and friends (interpretive control). A person with breast cancer might initiate a search for information on all aspects of her disease because feeling that she knows more about its future course makes it easier to cope (predictive control). Although the bias in Western culture is toward primary processes, secondary processes may facilitate adjustment when, in fact, the situation is objectively uncontrollable (Taylor et al., 1991).

The conditions under which primary control processes are most adaptive and those that favor secondary processes need to be examined. A step in that direction would be to assess the objective level of control a person has in a given situation as compared with the person's beliefs concerning his or her level of control. Measuring both the person's perceived control beliefs and the actual control that is available will allow us to predict more accurately which patients will experience enhanced adjustment and which patients will not. For instance, secondary control may be adaptive when a person has little objective control and the person perceives this accurately. Similarly, when control is objectively available and the person perceives it as such, primary control may be more adaptive.

Central and Consequence-Related Control

Another distinction is between central control, the belief that the event itself can be avoided or minimized (e.g., cancer can be cured), and consequence-related control, the belief that one can influence the impact of the event on other areas of life (e.g., prevent the cancer from adding stress to personal relationships) (Thompson et al., 1993). For example, a patient may correctly perceive the chemotherapy as being out of her control (it must happen) but judge that she can control its impact on her life. The patient might use medications to prevent the nausea from making her completely unavailable to her family, or she might take naps when other family members are out of the house so that she will have the energy to interact with them when they return. The patient can do little to avoid the chemotherapy, but she can exert some control over its consequences.

In studies of cancer and AIDS patients, Thompson and her colleagues found that consequence-related control was strongly related to less anxiety and depression, whereas they found no relationship or only a weak relationship between central control and psychological adjustment (Thompson, Nanni, & Levine, in press; Thompson et al., 1993). Similar results have been obtained with other samples of cancer and AIDS patients (Taylor & Collins, 1994; Taylor, Wayment, & Collins, 1993).

As with primary and secondary control processes, an assessment of central and consequence-related control allows for a more refined understanding of the role of perceived control in adjustment. Such refinements are necessary to untangle which components of control are essential to adjustment.

This section of the article has illustrated the trend toward specificity in assessing perceived control. This trend has taken us from general ideas concerning locus of control to more specific components of beliefs about control. For instance, to increase our understanding of the relationship between control and adjustment, we had to confront cultural beliefs in which primary processes were thought to be adaptive and secondary processes were thought to be maladaptive. A more accurate picture of the adaptiveness of these two processes may emerge when the objective level of control available to a person is compared to his or her beliefs about control in a specific situation. Similarly, distinguishing between control over the disease itself and control over the consequences of the disease has proved to be valuable in understanding the relationship between control and adjustment. Perhaps the conclusion to be derived from this section is that researchers will rarely err by being more specific about the components of control being assessed and by tailoring their measures for their specific populations.

CLINICAL APPLICATIONS

Although some people are able to maintain their sense of control as they go through stressful experiences such as being diagnosed with and treated for cancer, many others are not and could benefit from control-enhancing interventions. On the basis of a review of theories and research on control and control interventions, the first author proposed a model of the cognitive processes involved in judgments of perceived control that also serves as a schema for how to increase perceived control (Thompson, 1991).

In this scheme, perceived control can be enhanced by addressing eight questions regarding the identification of goals, controllable influences, alternative goals, current skills, ways to acquire skills, the accuracy of one's self-efficacy judgments, ways to increase self-efficacy, and the costs and benefits of asserting control. A sense of control is associated with knowing what you want, being able to identify workable ways to obtain it, switching to alternative goals when current goals are no longer attainable, being able to recognize your skills and abilities, knowing how to enhance those skills if necessary, and, finally, deciding when trying to assert control is worth the effort and when it is not. Problems and misperceptions in any of these areas can reduce perceptions of control. A therapist, support group leader, or social worker can use the scheme to help a client identify ways of thinking, self-perceptions, and misconceptions that may reduce a sense of autonomy and efficacy. For example, some people may have difficulty switching from an unattainable goal (e.g., avoiding medical treatment) to one that is feasible (e.g., maintaining equanimity while going through the treatment). The chance to think through what one wants and be exposed to the idea of recognizing attainable goals can help reduce feelings of helplessness.

CONCLUSION

There is no question that perceived control is relevant to the lives of those who are diagnosed with cancer. The loss of control experienced by patients has implications for their emotional well-being, and those who are able to restore or maintain feelings of mastery and autonomy are likely to have better psychological adjustment. Research on control processes for cancer patients has the promise of increasing our understanding of the adjustment process and developing interventions to promote the emotional well-being of those living with a diagnosis of cancer.

REFERENCES

Abramson, L. Y., Garber, J., & Seligman, M. E. P. (1980). Learned helplessness in humans: An attributional analysis. In Garber & Seligman (Eds.), *Human helplessness* (pp. 3-34). New York: Academic Press.

Affleck, G., Tennen, H., & Gershman, K. (1985). Cognitive adaptations to high-risk infants: The search for mastery, meaning, and protection from future harm. *American Journal of Mental Deficiency, 89,* 653-656.

Anastasi, A. (1976). *Psychological testing* (4th ed.). New York: Macmillan.

Avorn, J., & Langer, E. (1982). Induced disability in nursing home patients: A controlled trial. *Journal of the American Geriatrics Society, 30,* 397-400.

Bailey, K. D. (1993). *Methods of social research* (3rd ed.). New York: Free Press.

Bandura, A. (1977). Self-efficacy: Toward a unifying theory of behavioral change. *Psychological Review, 84,* 191-215.

Boggiano, A. K., & Katz, P. (1991). Maladaptive achievement patterns in students: The role of teachers' controlling strategies. *Journal of Social Issues, 47*(4), 35-51.

Burger, J. M. (1989). Negative reactions to increases in perceived personal control. *Journal of Personality & Social Psychology, 56,* 246-256.

Collins, B. E. (1974). Four components of the Rotter Internal-External Control scale: Belief in a difficult world, a just world, a predictable world, and a politically responsive world. *Journal of Personality & Social Psychology, 29,* 381-391.

Eccles, J. S., Buchanan, C. M., Flanagan, C., Fuligni, A., Midgley, C., & Yee, D. (1991). Control versus autonomy during early adolescence. *Journal of Social Issues, 47*(4), 53-67.

Ewart, C. K., Taylor, C. B., Reese, L. B., & DeBusk, R. F. (1983). Effects of early post-myocardial infarction exercise testing on self-perception and subsequent physical activity. *American Journal of Cardiology, 51,* 1076-1080.

Janoff-Bulman, R., & Frieze, I. H. (1983). A theoretical perspective for understanding reactions to victimization. *Journal of Social Issues, 39*(2), 1-17.

Lachman, M. E. (1991). Perceived control over memory aging: Developmental and intervention perspectives. *Journal of Social Issues, 47*(4), 159-175.

Lefcourt, H. M. (1991). Locus of control. In J. P. Robinson, P. R. Shaver, & L. S. Wrightsman (Eds.), *Measures of personality and social psychological attitudes* (pp. 413-499). San Diego, CA: Academic Press.

Marshall, G. N. (1991). A multidimensional analysis of internal health locus of control beliefs: Separating the wheat from the chaff? *Journal of Personality & Social Psychology, 61,* 483-491.

Miller, S. M. (1979). Controllability and human stress: Method, evidence, and theory. *Behavior Research & Therapy, 17,* 287-306.

Mirels, H. L. (1970). Dimensions of internal versus external control. *Journal of Consulting & Clinical Psychology, 15,* 266-279.

Nowicki, S., Jr., & Duke, M. P. (1983). The Nowicki-Strickland Life-span Locus of Control Scales: Construct validation. In H. M. Lefcourt (Ed.), *Research with the locus of control construct* (Vol. 2, pp. 9-51). New York: Academic Press.

Pearlin, L., & Schooler, C. (1978). The structure of coping. *Journal of Health & Social Behavior, 19,* 2-21.

Reich, J. W., & Zautra, A. J. (1990). Dispositional control beliefs and the consequences of a control-enhancing intervention. *Journal of Gerontology: Psychological Sciences, 45,* 46-51.

Reich, J. W., & Zautra, A. J. (1991). Experimental and measurement approaches to internal control in at-risk older adults. *Journal of Social Issues, 47*(4), 143-158.

Rodin, J. (1986). Health, control, and aging. In M. M. Baltes & P. B. Baltes (Eds.), *The psychology of aging and control* (pp. 139-166). Hillsdale, NJ: Lawrence Erlbaum.

Rodin, J. (1987). Personal control throughout the life course. In R. R. Abeles (Ed.), *Life-span perspectives and social psychology* (pp. 103-119). Hillsdale, NJ: Lawrence Erlbaum.

Rothbaum, F., Weisz, J., & Snyder, S. (1982). Changing the world and changing the self: A two-process model of perceived control. *Journal of Personality & Social Psychology, 42*, 5-37.

Rotter, J. B. (1966). Generalized expectancies for internal versus external control of reinforcement. *Psychological Monographs, 80*(1, Whole No. 609).

Seligman, M. E. P. (1975). *Helplessness*. New York: W. H. Freeman.

Seligman, M. E. P., Peterson, C., Kaslow, N. J., Tanenbaum, R. L., Alloy, L. B., & Abramson, L. Y. (1984). Attributional style and depressive symptoms among children. *Journal of Abnormal Psychology, 93*, 235-238.

Taylor, S. E. (1983). Adjustment to threatening events: A theory of cognitive adaptation. *American Psychologist, 38*, 1161-1173.

Taylor, S. E., & Collins, M. A. (In press). Medical treatment decision-making and buffers against regret. In D. Kahneman & G. Lowenstein (Eds.), *Anticipation and regret in health related decision-making*.

Taylor, S. E., Wayment, H. A., & Collins, M. A. (1993). Positive illusions and affect regulation. In D. M. Wegner & D. W. Pennebaker (Eds.), *Handbook of mental control* (pp. 325-343). Englewood Cliffs, NJ: Prentice-Hall.

Taylor, S. E., Helgeson, V. S., Reed, G. M., & Skokan, L. A. (1991). Self-generated feelings of control and adjustment to physical illness. *Journal of Social Issues, 47*(4), 91-109.

Thompson, S. C. (1981). A complex answer to a simple question: Will it hurt less if I can control it? *Psychological Bulletin, 90*, 89-101.

Thompson, S. C. (1991). Intervening to enhance perceptions of control. In C. R. Snyder & D. Forsyth (Eds.), *Handbook of social and clinical psychology* (pp. 607-623). New York: Pergamon Press.

Thompson, S. C. (1993). Naturally occurring perceptions of control: A model of bounded flexibility. In G. Weary, F. Gleicher, & K. Marsh (Eds.), *Control motivation and social cognition* (pp. 74-93). New York: Springer-Verlag.

Thompson, S. C., & Sobolew-Shubin, A. (1993). Overprotective relationships: A nonsupportive side of social networks. *Basic & Applied Social Psychology, 14*, 363-383.

Thompson, S. C., & Spacapan, S. (1991). Perceptions of control in vulnerable populations. *Journal of Social Issues, 47*(4), 1-21.

Thompson, S. C., Cheek, P. R., & Graham, M. A. (1988). The other side of perceived control: Disadvantages and negative effects. In S. Spacapan & S.

Oskamp (Eds.), *The social psychology of health* (pp. 69-93). Beverly Hills, CA: Sage Publications.

Thompson, S. C., Nanni, C., & Levine, A. (In press). Primary versus secondary and disease versus consequence-related control in HIV-positive men. *Journal of Personality & Social Psychology.*

Thompson, S. C., Sobolew-Shubin, A., Galbraith, M. E., Schwankovsky, L., & Cruzen, D. (1993). Maintaining perceptions of control: Finding perceived control in low-control circumstances. *Journal of Personality & Social Psychology, 64,* 293-304.

Wallston, K. A., & Wallston, B. S. (1981). Health locus of control scale. In H. M. Lefcourt (Ed.), *Research with the locus of control construct* (Vol. 1, pp. 189-243). New York: Academic Press.

Wallston, K. A., Wallston, B. S., & DeVellis, R. (1978). Development of the Multidimensional Health Locus of Control scale. *Health Education Monographs, 6,* 161-170.

Wortman, C. B., & Brehm, J. W. (1975). Responses to uncontrollable outcomes: An integration of reactance theory and the learned helplessness model. In L. Berkowitz (Ed.), *Advances in experimental social psychology* (Vol. 8, pp. 278-336). New York: Academic Press.

Exploring Relationships Between Cancer, Coping, and Mental Health

Michael Parle, MPsychol
Peter Maguire, MD

SUMMARY. The role that coping may play in mediating the psychological impact of cancer has been of considerable clinical and research interest. Despite this interest, however, the research has had several conceptual and methodological limitations that have resulted in weak and contradictory findings. The authors have used Lazarus and Folkman's transactional model of coping as a base from which to examine the influence of coping variables on the management of the demands of cancer. They discuss the measurement issues in researching this complex area, with reference to commonly cited instruments. In addition, they review recent research to identify the research questions and methodology that are most likely to be fruitful in exploring relationships between the demands of cancer, coping, and psychological impact. Suggestions are made for research that focuses on specific demands of cancer and incorporates different coping process variables more fully. *[Article copies are available from The Haworth Document Delivery Service: 1-800-342-9678.]*

Mr. Parle is a Research Clinical Psychologist, Cancer Research Campaign (CRC) Psychological Medicine Group, Stanley House, Christie Hospital, Wilmslow Road, Manchester M20 9BX, UK. Dr. Maguire is Director, CRC Psychological Medicine Group, and Senior Lecturer in Psychiatry, University of Manchester.

[Haworth co-indexing entry note]: "Exploring Relationships Between Cancer, Coping, and Mental Health." Parle, Michael, and Peter Maguire. Co-published simultaneously in the *Journal of Psychosocial Oncology* (The Haworth Medical Press, an imprint of The Haworth Press, Inc.) Vol. 13, No. 1/2, 1995, pp. 27-50; and: *Psychosocial Resource Variables in Cancer Studies: Conceptual and Measurement Issues* (ed: Barbara Curbow, and Mark R. Somerfield), The Haworth Medical Press, an imprint of The Haworth Press, Inc., 1995, pp. 27-50. *[Single or multiple copies of this article are available from The Haworth Document Delivery Service: 1-800-342-9678, 9:00 a.m. - 5:00 p.m. (EST)].*

Cancer patients are faced with multiple, diverse, and simultaneous demands. These demands may vary widely, from worry about prognosis to financial concerns arising from an inability to work. In addition, the impact of the demands may affect patients' mental health adversely and contribute to the high incidence of affective disorders that has been observed (Derogatis et al., 1983; Maguire et al., 1978). Consequently, researchers have attempted to establish what role coping plays in mediating between these demands, psychological adaptation, and progression of the disease.

Unfortunately, research on coping has been characterized by conceptual ambiguity and associated problems of measurement. Tunks and Bellissimo (1988, p. 171) reflected this in the following comment: "While it seems that *coping* has clinical utility it is very clear that this concept has significant . . . theoretical, semantic and scientific [limitations]." Recent reviews confirm that research into how patients cope with cancer has suffered from similar difficulties (Rowland, 1989; Somerfield & Curbow, 1992). Hence, the research findings have been weak and conflicting. As Lazarus (1993) notes, the commonly reported but oversimplified research designs are unlikely to unravel the relationship between coping and important outcomes. Thus, one must recognize that the assessment of coping is complex and requires rigorous measurement.

In this article, we provide a brief overview of coping and how the topic has been investigated in patients with cancer. We highlight the need to acknowledge that both coping and cancer are multifaceted and that measurement must take account of this. Moreover, the research questions must be precise to detect key relationships between coping, cancer, and different outcome variables.

ESTABLISHING A SCIENTIFIC DEFINITION OF COPING

The theoretical, semantic, and scientific limitations that Tunks and Bellissimo (1988) commented on are immediately evident when one attempts to define coping. In her review, Rowland (1989) reported several different ways in which coping has been defined in research studies. The diversity of definitions in a scientific context presents a number of impediments to effective research, especially in interpreting findings from studies that have adopted different meanings of the term.

From Rowland's useful summary (1989), we know that in its broadest sense, coping refers to adaptation to a demanding situation. There are differences of opinion about whether coping refers to *what* a person has done to adapt or *how well* he or she has adapted. Lazarus and Folkman (1984) attempted to reduce this conceptual ambiguity by discriminating the different elements associated with coping. We have used their model, which embraces four sets of variables–stimulus, appraisal, response, and outcome–as a base to clarify the scientific definition of coping and the variables associated with it (see Figure 1).

Within this framework of coping variables, the "stimulus for coping" refers to the demand or event that an individual is faced with. Appraisal variables include the individual's judgments about (1) whether the demand is potentially threatening (primary appraisal) and (2) what options exist to manage it (secondary appraisal). Response variables describe precisely what was done in an effort to manage the demand. Most commonly, the assessment of response variables is confined to questions about the type of response used and how often it was used. Additional dimensions associated with the response, such as the degree of skill with which it was performed, or motivational factors, including the amount of effort and degree of persistence, are neglected. Outcome variables assess the degree to which the responses used to manage the demand were successful. These variables can be classified as primary outcome variables, which Aldwin and Revenson (1987) described as *coping efficacy* (the extent to which the response resolved the demand), and secondary outcomes, or *coping effectiveness* (the effect of coping on mental or physical health).

The term coping, in its most widely cited scientific sense, refers to response variables or "constantly changing cognitive and behavioral efforts to manage specific external or internal demands that are appraised as taxing or exceeding the resources of the person" (Lazarus & Folkman, 1984, p. 141). This definition of coping is contingent upon appraisal but clearly separates measures of outcome. Importantly, Lazarus and Folkman (1984) argued that the coping responses involve purposeful rather than automatized activity. Defi-

FIGURE 1. Variables Associated with Different Models of Coping.

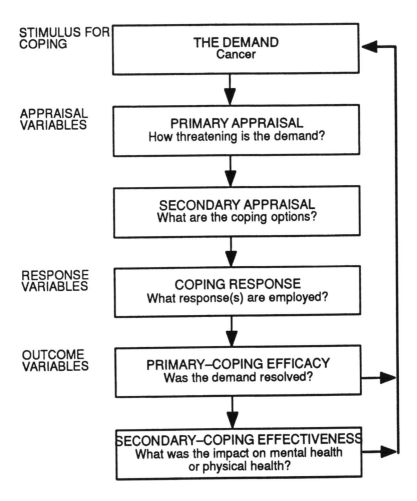

nitions of coping differ according to the specific variable referred to as "coping" and its relationships with the associated variables. Early behavioral and physiological models of coping made no reference to the role of appraisal. Instead, these models drew heavily from laboratory studies of animal behavior and explained coping as reflexive behaviors such as escape and avoidance in response to a noxious stimulus (Lazarus & Folkman, 1984). In other models, coping has been defined as outcome—the degree of success in adaptation—rather than as the type of response used (Lazarus & Folkman, 1984). More recently, Greer and Watson (1987) incorporated appraisal and response variables into a single variable: mental adjustment.

A diversity in theoretical models can promote important developments in understanding in areas of scientific research. We would argue, however, that coping is in need of semantic consolidation to ensure the construct validity of measures and improve the communication of findings. Within this scientific framework, researchers will be in a stronger position to debate the merits of different theoretical and empirical positions and their implications for patient care.

One primary debate has been whether coping is best understood as a trait or as a changing set of responses dependent on the specific character of the demand and the situation in which it occurs. Vaillant (1977), for example, conceptualized coping as defense mechanisms that are stable and generalized traits. In their transaction model of coping, Lazarus and Folkman (1984) argued that coping responses change constantly with ongoing appraisal and reappraisal of the specific situation. Their position, which emphasizes the importance of situational specificity in understanding and predicting behavior, is consistent with trends in measurement of a number of other psychological constructs. For example, the measurement of trait variables such as personality (Hampson, 1982) or global self-concept (Hansford & Hattie, 1982) have limited validity when predicting specific behavioral outcomes. In contrast, behavior- or situation-specific measures have proved to be more useful. In research on anxiety, self-efficacy ratings reliably predict the performance of relevant behaviors (Bandura, 1982, 1988), whereas in self-concept research, the development of specific measures such as academic self-concept has produced stronger and more consistent findings than have global measures in relation to academic performance and its impact on adolescents (e.g., Marsh, 1990).

Despite the limitations of the trait approach, the type of coping response used in a specified situation is likely to be accounted for by a complex interaction of personal and situational variables. Accordingly, different, more recently developed cognitive models of coping use the transactional model as a basis but have attempted to incorporate both generalized (coping style) and situational factors to explain an individual's coping behavior (e.g., Carver, Scheier, & Weintraub, 1989; Miller, Combs, & Stoddard, 1989).

CANCER AS THE STIMULUS FOR COPING

Cancer, like coping, does not represent a unitary variable, but it includes a broad and diverse range of demands (Dunkel-Schetter et al., 1992). Yet, surprisingly little consideration has been paid to how cancer might be assessed as a stimulus for coping. Coping with cancer has been investigated at various levels–from coping with the generalized experience of having cancer to coping with specific demands such as the side effects of treatment. A study that focuses on the measurement of coping with a single specific demand may not be markedly different from coping research in fields other than oncology. A key difficulty facing this area of research, though, is understanding how to assess coping validly with the generalized experience of cancer.

Two methods are commonly used in generalized assessments of coping with cancer. One approach considers cancer at a global level, represented as a unitary variable (see Figure 2). This is essentially a trait approach, which assumes that the different demands associated with cancer are sufficiently similar to permit aggregation and that patients would use similar responses across different demands. We know of no reliable data that support these assumptions. The global approach also fails to establish which specific demands a patient has appraised as threatening and is attempting to cope with. The implications of the global approach are illustrated by a patient who has cervical cancer. She may simultaneously face fears of recurrence, concerns about her self-esteem, sexual difficulties because of the anatomical effect of treatment, and concerns about needing extended time off from work. In answer to questions about how she is coping with cancer, she may think selectively about one of these concerns, leaving the others unrepresented, or provide a mixed answer that attempts to aggregate all her concerns, which makes it difficult to disentangle her coping efforts. Attempts to make meaningful comparisons with other patients' coping is likely to be even more haphazard.

The second dominant approach has been to sample coping behav-

FIGURE 2. An Example of How Cancer Demands Can Be Represented at Global and More Specific Levels of Measurement.

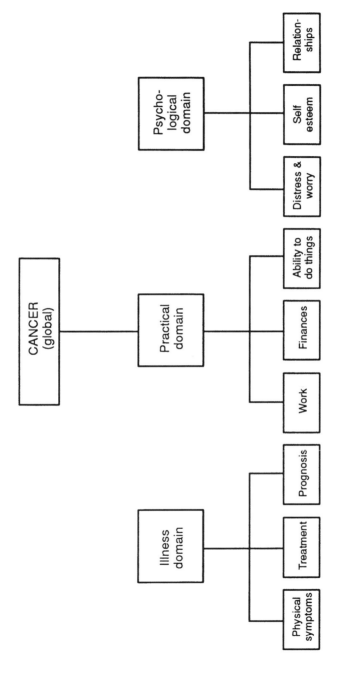

ior by asking patients how they have coped with one recent demand they appraised as stressful. This approach allows more detailed information to be elicited about their coping efforts regarding that demand. Difficulties arise when this sample of coping is interpreted as representative of coping with cancer. The shortcomings of this approach are evident when between-patient comparisons of coping are made across an uncontrolled range of demands. A patient's responses to feelings of disfigurement can be compared with another patient's coping responses to financial concerns. Further shortcomings arise when one assumes that the single sample of coping with any cancer demand is representative of how a patient manages similar demands at other times or that this sample represents the skills required to negotiate multiple demands simultaneously.

Coping research based on the global assessment of cancer demands and that based on a single case example provide important information but require additional validation if they are to be considered as representative of coping with cancer. The assessment of coping in response to multiple concerns should provide more reliable samples of coping from which to generalize results.

MEASUREMENT

We will now review a number of instruments with the primary aims of illustrating what coping variables the instruments assess and the type of research questions they might answer best in studies of coping with cancer.

Ways of Coping Questionnaire

One of the original and widely reported instruments used to measure coping is the Ways of Coping Questionnaire (WCQ), a self-report questionnaire that assesses the type of coping responses that subjects use to manage a recent stressful situation (Folkman & Lazarus, 1985; Lazarus & Folkman, 1984). Each item describes a coping response that the subject rates according to the extent that he or she used that strategy ("Not used" to "Used a great deal"). Additional questions can be asked about what was at stake in the situation (primary appraisal) and what coping options the subject considered (secondary appraisal). The WCQ can yield information about how often each response was used; the overall number of response strategies used; and the type of response, summarized as either problem or emotion focused; or one of eight statistically derived categories. The statistically derived categories have been criticized, however, as being based on an unstable factor structure (Endler & Parker, 1990).

Although the WCQ attempts to measure coping responses separately from other variables such as appraisal or outcome, it has been criticized because of the limited range of responses assessed (Carver, Scheier, & Weintraub, 1989), particularly with regard to cancer demands. Two research groups in the United Kingdom attempted to modify the instrument for use with breast cancer patients (Cooper & Faragher, 1992; Jarrett et al., 1992). Jarrett et al. (1992) eliminated 13 items they regarded as inappropriate and produced a 53-item questionnaire, which they tested empirically with 153 breast cancer patients. The factor structure of the revised questionnaire did not correspond to the original WCQ coping factors. However, this result should not be overinterpreted, given the reduced pool of items and the marginal subject-to-item ratio (Stevens, 1986). Jarrett et al. reported that the revised questionnaire provided a quick means of assessing coping responses without observer bias; however, some patients had conceptual difficulty reflecting on the responses they used, especially those related to avoidance. Cooper and Faragher (1992, 1993) modified the WCQ for use with women presenting for investigation of breast symptoms. Those authors selected the 36 most frequently endorsed strategies by patient volunteers in a previous study for use in a prospective study of 2,163 women who presented for breast cancer screening or investigation. They reported that their modified version yielded five interpretable factors and that the questionnaire as a whole had reasonable internal consistency (Cronbach's alpha = .789), but no reliability data were reported for their five subscales.

COPE Questionnaire

The COPE questionnaire is another self-report questionnaire that assesses coping responses but differs from the WCQ in its taxonomy of coping responses (Carver, Scheier, & Weintraub, 1989). The taxonomy of coping responses has been derived from both a theoretical perspective and from other questionnaires. Both situational and dispositional versions of the questionnaire have been developed. The psychometric properties of the instrument are modest, but they appear to have room for improvement in the factor structure (Carver, Sheier, & Weintrub, 1989). In a recent study with breast cancer patients, Carver et al. (1993) reported that modifications were necessary in several subscales because of difficulties with reliability. Additional independent assessment of this new instrument would be helpful to determine how well it generalizes across study populations. A further development by Carver et al. (1993) is the concurrent use of the COPE and a generalized appraisal measure, the Life Orientation Test (LOT) (Scheier & Carver, 1985). The LOT, a brief scale designed to measure optimism and pessimism, may provide a useful measure of subjects' expectations regarding the outcome of coping in novel or ambiguous situations.

The WCQ and similar questionnaires have often been used in cross-sectional studies to assess a single sample of coping behavior from an uncontrolled range of demands. Therefore, they are subject to the limitations we have described when between-patient comparisons are made on the basis of responses to different types of demands. To a large extent, these limitations can be overcome with a more judicious application of these questionnaires. For example, Dunkel-Schetter et al. (1992) addressed the problem, in part, by confining their investigation to coping responses to one of four common cancer demands from which patients could select one that they had appraised as stressful. Such an approach may allow the emergence of more reliable findings.

Mental Adjustment to Cancer Scale

The Mental Adjustment to Cancer (MAC) scale represents an alternative approach to the measurement of coping with cancer (Greer & Watson, 1987; Watson et al., 1988). First, this self-report questionnaire represents cancer as a global variable. Second, rather than measuring coping variables separately, the MAC incorporates both appraisal (e.g., "I see my illness as a challenge") and coping responses ("I am trying to get as much information as I can about cancer") into one coping variable described as a "mental adjustment style" (Greer & Watson, 1987). Questions about coping outcomes appear to be included in the mental adjustment variable as well ("Since my cancer diagnosis I now realize how precious life is and I am making the most of it").

The MAC was validated with cancer patients in the United Kingdom and was found to have reasonable psychometric support. It was originally reported to yield five adjustment styles: anxious preoccupation, helplessness, fatalism, avoidance, and fighting spirit (Greer & Watson, 1987), but the Avoidance subscale has not been reported in later research (Watson et al., 1991). Much of the validation has been based on correlations with scores on the Hospital Anxiety and Depression Scale (HADS), a measure of mental health (Zigmond & Snaith, 1983). On the basis of early data, the correlations between the MAC subscales and the HADS anxiety and depression scores were generally small (.19 to -.29) except for the relationship between the Anxious Preoccupation subscale and the HADS Anxiety subscale ($r = .48$) (Watson et al., 1988). Stronger relationships have since been observed between helplessness and depression and anxiety ($r = .40$ and $r = 44$, respectively) and between anxious preoccupation and depression and anxiety ($r = .43$ and $r = .60$, respectively) (Watson et al., 1991). The MAC is easy to administer and is intended for use in busy clinics. However, because it is based on an aggregated measure of appraisal, coping, and outcome variables and a global assessment of cancer, it sacrifices detail about specific problems a patient may be experiencing. Because of the MAC's strong emphasis on helplessness and fighting spirit, refining the instrument as a global cancer-appraisal scale similar in purpose to the LOT may be more useful. In this capacity, it could be applied more strategically with other measures of coping responses and coping outcomes.

Measure of Psychological Adjustment

Dunn et al. (1993) have developed a measure of "psychological adjustment" to cancer that is derived from a scale used with diabetic patients. The authors report that a thorough validation procedure ensures that the scale is appropriate for use with cancer patients and have found that the measure has encouraging psychometric properties in applications. This questionnaire provides an omnibus "psychological adjustment" variable intended to measure functional outcomes of coping, but instead it appears to incorporate elements of appraisal, coping response, and coping outcomes. This is reflected in the six factors extracted in the questionnaire: stigma about having cancer, minimization, cooperative dependence (with the medical profession), cancer severity/hope (impact of the disease and hope for cure), responsibility (for treatment), and avoidance/denial. The difficulty with questionnaires such as this measure of psychological adjustment or the MAC is that they appear to have sacrificed discrimination between key psychological variables with little gain in detail about cancer. Hence, they are in danger of falling between being a validated measure of mental health such as the HADS and a detailed questionnaire such as the WCQ, which assesses coping responses. Therefore, to date, no self-report questionnaire is available that maintains specificity in the assessment of coping process variables as well as assesses cancer-specific demands.

Semistructured Interviews

A further approach to measuring coping involves the use of semistructured interviews. Both Jarrett et al. (1992) and Somerfield and Curbow (1992) discussed this method of assessment. As Jarrett and colleagues commented, the semistructured interview can be especially useful to help patients clarify the coping responses they used and can be more sensitive to "avoidance" or responses that can be described as "denial."

We recently used a semistructured interview to investigate the concerns and coping responses of newly diagnosed cancer patients. In the interview, patients' specific concerns arising from their diagnosis were elicited. The patients were then asked about the main coping response they used for each concern they had appraised as worrisome. Finally, the degree of resolution achieved by their coping responses was assessed. Interviews were tape recorded, and the patients' coping responses were subsequently coded into 1 of 31 cognitive and behavioral responses that also allowed the rating of negative responses such as "feeling helpless" and "do nothing." The coding manual for these coping responses was derived from a series of studies with lymphoma patients (Devlen, 1984) and has been found to produce acceptable interrater reliability ($r = .84$) (Devlen, Phillips, & Maguire, 1991).

The main advantages of the semistructured interview are that it allows the assessment of coping with multiple demands and, like other interview schedules, elicits greater information about how patients actually responded to each demand. In addition, the interview format allows the assessment of a far greater variety of responses than is possible with a standardized self-report questionnaire. The measurement of the degree of success in resolving a concern (coping efficacy) also can help to identify factors that may contribute to the successful performance of a response, but these factors are ignored in existing self-report measures of coping responses.

One disadvantage of the interview schedule in its current format is that only one coping response is elicited for each concern. In addition, the schedule has received some criticism because the classification of coping strategies cannot be reduced to a few factors. This may suggest that these coping strategies are distinct and worth measuring separately. Another disadvantage is that the interview is more time consuming, both to administer and to code, than are standardized self-report instruments.

In summary, the instruments used to explore the relationships between coping and cancer leave room for improvement. We have reviewed several instruments and have attempted to indicate the circumstances in which they may be most appropriate. When deciding which of these or other similar instruments to use, one needs to consider what coping variables are relevant to the research questions. The purpose may be to assess coping responses to a specific event (e.g., an invasive medical procedure), or it may be to investigate the coping process more thoroughly, including appraisal and efficacy and generalized coping outcome such as mental health. Practical issues such as the resources available to administer, code, and analyze the results also need to be considered. A semistructured interview, administered and coded by trained interviewers, can provide high-quality information. However, if this procedure is not feasible, a self-report measure might be preferable.

RECENT RESEARCH

In this section, we will discuss recent research on coping responses and the demands of cancer within three contexts: (1) studies that have focused on the measurement of coping-efficacy outcomes (resolution of the demand itself), (2) studies that have examined relationships between coping responses and coping-effectiveness outcomes (mental or physical health or both), and (3) studies that have used primary or secondary appraisal to clarify the role these variables may have in the process of coping with cancer.

Coping Efficacy

Coping efficacy is often overlooked in measures of coping outcomes despite its clinical and theoretical importance. The resolution of demands can have immediate benefits for cancer patients. The success of responses undertaken to relieve pain, clarify information, or improve the level of support can have a marked impact on patients' immediate quality of life. A patient's inability to resolve a demand also may contribute to subsequent poor mental health through the cumulative strain of ongoing demands. In addition, the impact of negative feedback from unsuccessful coping efforts on expectancies regarding outcome may inhibit the quality of subsequent coping responses.

Studies designed to assess coping efficacy outcomes have certain methodological advantages. By limiting the scope of a study to investigate coping variables that promote the resolution of a specific demand, the researcher is able to exercise greater experimental control and use more thorough measurement procedures. These research designs also provide more opportunity to identify the factors that may influence the success of a coping response. This is illustrated by research on coping with diagnostic tests and treatments such as radiotherapy (Peterson, 1989).

A number of these studies have evaluated the success of relaxation strategies designed to help patients cope with different medical procedures. For example, Gattuso, Litt, and Fitzgerald (1992) reported that the success of muscle relaxation as a coping strategy to relieve the distress and discomfort associated with gastroscopy improved significantly with the use of techniques that enhanced self-efficacy, which reinforced the importance of secondary appraisal to the coping process. Miller, Combs, and Stoddard (1989) reviewed a number of other studies in which relaxation techniques have been taught as a coping response for chemotherapy. They found that muscle relaxation techniques reduced posttreatment nausea and vomiting, although the efficacy of this coping response varied across studies according to the degree of support from the therapist and the use of complementary cognitive skills such as guided imagery and, in the case of anticipatory nausea, systematic desensitization.

These different studies highlight just how much variation can occur in the use of one type of coping response. The degree of success of relaxation as a coping response varied considerably and depended on factors such as the level of self-efficacy, the extent to which the skill had been learned competently, and the appropriateness of the response to the demand (differing even between anticipatory and posttreatment nausea). Therefore, specificity in assessment is important in the evaluation of a coping response. Because of this variation in the success of a coping response, researchers, again, must be cautious about interpreting assessments that ask no more than the frequency with which a patient used the response to cope with cancer.

Coping Effectiveness

Investigations of the mental and physical health outcomes of coping have produced contradictory findings and must be viewed critically. Watson et al. (1988) noted in their review of the literature that denial had been variously reported to be predictive of good and poor mental health. In a longitudinal study, Greer (1991) reported that fighting spirit and denial were predictive of survival for English breast cancer patients at 5, 10, and 15 years. His findings were replicated on an American sample. In their research on women undergoing screening and diagnostic tests for breast cancer, Cooper and Faragher (1992, 1993) used a modified version of the WCQ and found that a coping response they described as denial was associated with malignancy, whereas anger was related to a benign diagnosis. Using the COPE measure, Carver et al. (1993) reported that acceptance, sense of humor, and religion were protective of breast cancer patients' mental health, whereas denial and disengagement predicted distress.

Little sense can be made of these discrepant findings until the wide variation resulting from measurement and methodological factors is eliminated. For example, denial, identified in the research just described as both promoting and inhibiting mental and physical health, has been based on different items assessed in response to equally diverse types of demands. Carver et al. (1993) based their results on a two-item denial subscale that included items such as "I refuse to believe this has happened" in response to any single recent stressful situation. Cooper and Faragher (1992, 1993) labeled an 11-item factor as "denial" with items such as "I get on with work, keep busy, do some housework" also in response to a recent stressful life event. Greer (1991) identified the use of denial from patients' avoidance and minimization responses disclosed in a semistructured interview. Hence, it is doubtful that consistent results will emerge across studies until greater methodological rigor is used. Comparable and more guarded use of terminology such as denial will help this process. Moreover, instead of attempting to ask an open question, "Does denial work?" more strategic research that investigates the situations in which denial helps adaptation and situations in which denial inhibits it may be more fruitful.

The Role of Appraisal

Perhaps the most consistent coping relationship observed in cancer research has been the one between helplessness or pessimism and poor mental and physical health (Carver et al., 1993; Greer, 1991; Stein, Hermanson, & Spiegel, 1993; Watson et al., 1991). Similar findings have been reported in other areas of physical illness such as research on chronic pain (Jensen et al., 1991). A relationship also has been observed between optimism and fighting spirit and positive outcomes of coping, although the relationship with fighting spirit is not as strong (Watson et al., 1991). Helplessness and pessimism, more accurately understood as appraisal variables rather than response variables, reinforce Lazarus and Folkman's emphasis (1984) that appraisal variables are integral to the coping process.

The key role of appraisal variables in coping has become apparent in social and clinical psychological research. In his work on self-efficacy, Bandura (1982, 1988) demonstrated that appraisals have important motivational, behavioral, and affective consequences for the coping process. Bandura found that people with high self-efficacy were more likely to initiate coping responses, expend more effort, persist in the face of difficulty, and experience less distress than were their less confident counterparts. Gattuso, Litt, and Fitzgerald's study (1992) on the role of self-efficacy and the success of relaxation techniques in patients undergoing gastroscopy provides some support for Bandura's findings. Similarly, Felton and Revenson (1984) described a "mutually reinforcing cycle" in which those who initially felt more threatened and distressed in a situation were more likely to make maladaptive coping responses that exacerbated their problems. In their study, Dunkel-Schetter et al. (1992) found that certain responses such as escape and avoidance proved to be associated with greater appraisals of stress. Their findings indicated, however, that a number of other contextual variables such as availability of social support are likely to be involved.

In cognitive theories of psychopathology, some have argued that individual differences in primary and secondary appraisals are key factors in the onset and maintenance of anxiety and depressive disorders. According to Kendall (1992), adaptive or healthy thinking involves an ability to filter out numerous possibilities of threat present in any environment to a level that is manageable. This process was illustrated in a social psychology study by Croyle (1992). Subjects who were told they had tested positive to a (fictitious) health threat gave it significantly lower severity ratings than did those who were given a negative test result. According to Beck and colleagues (e.g., Beck & Clark, 1988; Beck & Emery, 1985), individuals who are vulnerable to mental health problems such as anxiety and depression are less able to appraise situations in a protective manner. Instead, they systematically process information about the situation in such a way that the situation is perceived to be highly threatening; at the same time, they underestimate their coping options.

Recent findings from a prospective study of psychological reactions to a malignant cervical diagnosis suggest that maladaptive coping may be initiated by selective attentional processes that influence appraisal (MacLeod & Hagan, 1992). MacLeod and Hagan used the Stroop Color-naming Test that measures the degree to which subjects are distracted from a simple computer-based task (naming the color that a word is presented in on a screen) by the degree of threat implied by the content of the word (e.g., "disease" as opposed to "leisure"). They found that the degree to which the women were distracted from the color-naming task by high-threat words (assessed before they had their colposcopy) significantly predicted distress measured eight weeks after diagnosis. These results suggest that vulnerable individuals focus more on possible threat stimuli in a situation, whereas others are able to distract themselves. Therefore, psychological vulnerabilities such as a bias in attention toward possible threatening stimuli may precede the cancer diagnosis and have a significant impact on a patient's process of coping with cancer.

We have recently found empirical support for the complex effects of appraisal on coping responses and coping outcomes in our own research. In preliminary results from a prospective study of affective disorders among cancer patients (Parle, Jones, & Maguire, 1994), appraisal, coping response, and coping efficacy were all found to be significant predictors of subsequent affective disorders. Patients were interviewed soon after diagnosis and asked what cancer-related concerns they had appraised as worrying, what they had done to manage these concerns, and how successful their responses had been. Patients who reported more concerns, gave the concerns higher ratings of severity, felt helpless or believed they could do nothing to manage, and rated their coping efforts as less successful were at greater risk for subsequent affective disorder. Moreover, in multivariate analyses, only appraisal of concerns (the amount of worry reported for 14 cancer-related concerns) and coping efficacy (patients' ratings of the degree to which they had resolved their concerns) remained significant. The type of coping response ceased to be predictive when the effectiveness of appraisal and performance were taken into account.

In summary, the recent literature on coping has generated more questions than it has resolved. This is particularly true of research that has attempted to make links between coping responses and mental health without heeding appraisal variables or the extent to which demands are resolved. The most fruitful results reported recently have come from three areas. First, experimental studies on the efficacy of particular strategies for dealing with specific concerns provide information that may affect patients' quality of life. Second, research studies such as Dunkel-Schetter et al.'s (1992) have demonstrated how greater theoretical and methodological rigor can be applied when investigating the complex relationships between personal characteristics, medical variables, appraisal, and coping responses. Third, interesting research such as MacLeod and Hagan's (1992) has illustrated the importance of appraisal variables on coping outcomes. To date, no individual coping response has proved to be consistently protective of psychological distress or progression of disease. Appraisal factors such as hopelessness or pessimism have received much more consistent support. The importance of these appraisal variables is illustrated in their effects on the selection, initiation, performance, and persistence of any coping response. Overall, examining the type of coping response alone, especially with regard to its influence on secondary outcomes, has proved to be inadequate.

LOOKING FORWARD

The potential contribution of an understanding of coping to the clinical care of cancer patients is high but has yet to be fulfilled. One reason is the overemphasis on the investigation of relationships between the type of coping responses used for a limited sample of demands and secondary outcomes such as mental health. This approach has largely ignored the contribution of other coping variables and the complexity of cancer. To realize the full contribution of coping research to clinical care, attention must be paid to the characteristics of cancer, appraisal variables, coping responses, and coping efficacy.

Characteristics of the cancer experience. The validity of research on coping necessitates some consideration of the stimulus for coping. Patients with cancer face many and varying demands that they must attempt to meet. Making a global assessment of how a patient is coping or examining only a single sample of coping with those demands does not do justice to the complexity of the cancer experience and is unlikely to yield robust information about the link between appraisal, coping responses, and longer-term outcomes concerning mental and physical health.

Appraisal variables. Although Lazarus and Folkman (1984) emphasized the importance of appraisal variables, most research on coping with cancer has made only passing references to them. Later research has supported cognitive models of psychopathology in which appraisal variables have been implicated as rendering certain individuals vulnerable to affective disorders (Bandura, 1988; Beck & Clark, 1988). Because these results have particular relevance for an understanding of the entire coping process, they deserve a more thorough investigation.

Coping responses. We have emphasized the need to assess how patients perform their coping responses rather than merely state what responses they use and how often. These performance variables include factors that affect the level of skill and competence exhibited as well as the degree of persistence and effort in carrying out any specific strategy. For example, one has no reason to assume that relaxation techniques performed poorly or inappropriately are as effective as relaxation techniques performed competently. Yet, much coping research rests on this assumption. Similarly, the successful use of "acceptance" may be associated with a sense of relief, reduction of symptoms of anxiety and depression, and a reappraisal of concerns. When acceptance fails to work, it could lead to much greater frustration, tension, and despondency.

At present, only semistructured interviews conducted by trained raters are able to separate out mediating variables that are likely to influence the success of a coping response. Some research evidence indicates that this approach can be used to good effect. Detailed cognitive behavioral analysis of existing coping responses has led to the improvement of previously intractable problems such as persistent symptoms of schizophrenia (Tarrier et al., 1992). In the context of cancer, similar techniques appear to have been overlooked in favor of elaborate taxonomies that emphasize the content and frequency of coping responses rather than their effectiveness. However, adopting common definitions is important to ensure that frequently used terms such as denial are used validly and reliably before one uses meta-analyses to summarize these studies and comes to unhelpful conclusions.

Coping efficacy. Considerable progress can be made through research that focuses on the most common demands placed on cancer patients: for example, how they respond to bad news, manage the inevitable uncertainty about their prognosis, and deal with side effects of their illness and treatment. Research into what variables promote the resolution of these concerns is necessary to determine the effects of the coping process on secondary outcome variables. Whether patients who fail to resolve their concerns or believe they have been unsuccessful will maintain positive levels of mental health is doubtful. In addition, information obtained from well-controlled longitudinal studies on coping efficacy may provide a more solid basis for deciding what variables are most salient in the coping process. Factors that may determine whether patients resolve their concerns should receive special emphasis.

CONCLUSION

The measurement of coping with cancer faces many challenges. Although Lazarus and Folkman's model of coping is commonly endorsed, their recommendations have rarely been translated into practice. Current research is characterized by methods of measurement and research questions that confuse appraisal, coping, and outcome variables or overrepresent the explanatory potential of coping responses. These methods and questions do so by trying to establish a direct link between the type of response alone, from a single sample of coping behavior, to indicators of coping effectiveness. Robust findings will result only if more attention is paid to strategic and theoretically substantiated research questions. This approach is likely to increase research options rather than inhibit them.

REFERENCES

Aldwin, C. M., & Revenson, T. A. (1987). Does coping help? A reexamination of the relation between coping and mental health. *Journal of Personality & Social Psychology, 53*, 337-348.

Bandura, A. (1982). The self and mechanisms in human agency. *American Psychologist, 37*, 122-147.

Bandura, A. (1988). Self-efficacy conception of anxiety. *Anxiety Research, 1*, 77-98.

Beck, A. T., & Clark, D. A. (1988). Anxiety and depression: An information processing perspective. *Anxiety Research, 1*, 23-36.

Beck, A. T., & Emery, G. (1985). *Anxiety disorders and phobias: A cognitive perspective*. New York: Basic Books.

Carver, C. S., Scheier, M. F., & Weintraub, J. K. (1989). Assessing coping strategies: A theoretically based approach. *Journal of Personality & Social Psychology, 56*, 267-283.

Carver, S. C., Pozo, C., Harris, S. D., Noriega, V., Scheier, M. F., Robinson, D. S., Ketcham, A. S., Moffat, F. L., Jr., & Clark, K. C. (1993). How coping mediates the effect of optimism on distress: A study of women with early stage breast cancer. *Journal of Personality & Social Psychology, 65*, 375-390.

Cooper, C. L., & Faragher, E. B. (1992). Coping strategies and breast disorders/cancer. *Psychological Medicine, 22*, 447-455.

Cooper, C. L., & Faragher, E. B. (1993). Psychosocial stress and breast cancer: The interrelationship between stress events, coping strategies and personality. *Psychological Medicine, 23*, 653-662.

Croyle, R. T. (1992). Appraisal of health threats: Cognition, motivation and social comparison. *Cognitive Therapy & Research, 16*, 165-182.

Derogatis, L. R., Morrow, G. R., Fetting, J., Penman, D., Piasetsky, S., Schmale, A. M., Henrichs, M., & Carnicke, C. L. M., Jr. (1983). The prevalence of psychiatric disorders amongst cancer patients. *Journal of the American Medical Association, 249*, 751-757.

Devlen, J. (1984). Psychological and social aspects of Hodgkin's disease and non-Hodgkin's lymphoma. Doctoral thesis, University of Manchester, Manchester, UK.

Devlen, J., Phillips, P., & Maguire, P. (1991). Development of a classification of coping strategies. Unpublished manuscript, Cancer Research Campaign Psychological Medicine Group.

Dunkel-Schetter, C., Feinstein, L., Taylor, S., & Falke, R. (1992). Patterns of coping with cancer. *Health Psychology, 11*, 79-87.

Dunn, S. M., Patterson, P., Butow, P. N., Smartt, H. H., McCarthy, W. H., & Tattersall, H. N. (1993). Cancer by another name: A randomized trial of the effects of euphemism and uncertainty in communicating with cancer patients. *Journal of Clinical Oncology, 11*, 989-996.

Endler, N. S., & Parker, J. D. A. (1990). Multidimensional assessment of coping: A critical evaluation. *Journal of Personality & Social Psychology, 58*, 844-854.

Felton, B. J., & Revenson, T. A. (1984). Coping with a chronic illness: A study of illness controllability and the influence of coping strategies on psychological adjustment. *Journal of Consulting & Clinical Psychology, 52*, 343-353.

Folkman, S., & Lazarus, R. S. (1985). If it changes it must be a process: A study of emotion and coping during three stages of a college examination. *Journal of Personality & Social Psychology, 48*, 150-170.

Gattuso, S. M., Litt, M., Fitzgerald, T. E. (1992). Coping with gastrointestinal endoscopy: Self-efficacy enhancement and coping style. *Journal of Consulting & Clinical Psychology, 60*, 133-139.

Greer, S. (1991). Psychological response to cancer and survival. *Psychological Medicine, 21*, 43-49.

Greer, S., & Watson, M. (1987). Mental adjustment to cancer: Its measurement and prognostic importance. *Cancer Surveys, 6*, 439-453.

Hampson, S. E. (1982). *The construction of personality.* Boston: Routledge & Kegan Paul.

Hansford, B. C., & Hattie, J. A. (1982). The relationship between self and achievement/performance measures. *Review of Educational Research, 52*, 123-142.

Jarrett, S. R., Ramirez, A. J., Richards, M. A., & Weinman, J. (1992). Measuring coping in breast cancer. *Journal of Psychosomatic Research, 36*, 593-602.

Jensen, M. P., Turner, J. A., Romano, J. M., & Karoly, P. (1991). Coping with chronic pain: A critical review of the literature. *Pain, 47*, 249-283.

Kendall, P. C. (1992). Healthy thinking. *Behavior Therapy, 23*, 1-11.

Lazarus, R. S. (1993). Coping theory and research: Past, present and future. *Psychosomatic Medicine, 55*, 234-247.

Lazarus, R. S., & Folkman, S. (1984). *Stress, appraisal and coping.* New York: Springer Publishing.

MacLeod, C., & Hagan, R. (1992). Individual differences in the selective processing of threatening information and emotional responses to a stressful life event. *Behavior Research & Therapy, 30*, 151-161.

Maguire, G. P., Lee, E. G., Bevington, D. J., Kuchemann, C. S., Crabtree, R. J., & Cornell, C. E. (1978). Psychiatric problems in the first year after mastectomy. *British Medical Journal, 1*, 963-965.

Marsh, H. (1990). A multidimensional, hierarchical model of self-concept: Theoretical and empirical justification. *Educational Psychology Review, 2*, 77-172.

Miller, S. M., Combs, C., & Stoddard, E. (1989). Information, coping and control in patients undergoing surgery and stressful medical procedures. In A. Steptoe & A. Appeals (Eds.), *Stress, personal control and health.* Chichester, England: John Wiley & Sons.

Parle, M., Jones, B., & Maguire, P. (1994). Maladaptive coping and affective disorders amongst cancer patients. Manuscript under review.

Peterson, L. (1989). Special series: Coping with medical illness and medical procedures. *Journal of Consulting & Clinical Psychology, 57*, 331-332.

Rowland, J. H. (1989). Intrapersonal resources: Coping. In J. C. Holland & Rowland (Eds.), *Handbook of Psychooncology: Psychological care of the patient with cancer.* New York: Oxford University Press.

Scheier, M. F., & Carver, C. S. (1985). Optimism, coping and health: Assessment and implications of generalized outcome expectancies. *Health Psychology, 4*, 219-247.

Somerfield, M., & Curbow, B. (1992). Methodological issues and research strategies in the study of coping with cancer. *Social Science & Medicine, 34*, 1203-1261.

Stein, S., Hermanson, K., & Spiegel, D. (1993). New directions in psycho-oncology. *Current Opinion in Psychiatry, 6*, 838-846.

Stevens, J. (1986). *Applied multivariate statistics for the social sciences*. Hillsdale, NJ: Lawrence Erlbaum.

Tarrier, N., Sharpe, L., Beckett, R., Harwood, S., Baker, A., & Yusopoff, L. (1992). A trial of two cognitive behavioral methods of treating drug resistant psychotic symptoms in schizophrenic patients: II. Treatment specific changes in coping and problem solving. *Social Psychiatry & Psychiatric Epidemiology, 28*, 5-10.

Tunks, E., & Bellissimo, A. (1988). Coping with the coping concept: A brief comment. *Pain, 34*, 171-174.

Vaillant, G. E. (1977). *Adaptation to life*. Boston: Little, Brown.

Watson, M., Greer, S., Young, J., Inayat, Q., Burgess, C., & Robertson, B. (1988). Development of a questionnaire of adjustment to cancer: The MAC scale. *Psychological Medicine, 18*, 203-209.

Watson, M., Greer, S., Rowden, L., Gorman, C., Robertson, B., Bliss, J. M., & Tunmore, R. T. (1991). Relationships between emotional control, adjustment to cancer and depression and anxiety in breast cancer patients. *Psychological Medicine, 21*, 51-57.

Zigmond, A., & Snaith, R. (1983). The Hospital and Anxiety Depression Scale. *Acta Psychiatrica Scandinavia, 67*, 361-370.

Religion and Spirituality as Resources for Coping with Cancer

Richard A. Jenkins, PhD
Kenneth I. Pargament, PhD

SUMMARY. Studies of coping with cancer have often included variables concerned with religion or spirituality. Unfortunately, the variables chosen have generally had limited salience for the overall coping process and limited usefulness for the development of clinical interventions. Despite these drawbacks, existing research suggests that religious and spiritual coping may have positive impacts on cancer patients' adjustment, and some evidence exists that suggests ways in which religion and spirituality may fit into the coping process. Considerations in the selection of better measures and more useful conceptualizations of religious or spiritual coping are offered as well as suggestions for more beneficial assessments of religious or spiritual functioning in clinical contexts. *[Article copies are available from The Haworth Document Delivery Service: 1-800-342-9678.]*

Dr. Jenkins is Research Assistant Professor, Uniformed Services University of the Health Sciences, Bethesda, MD, and Senior Staff Scientist, Behavioral Prevention Program, Henry M. Jackson Foundation for the Advancement of Military Medicine, Rockville, MD. Dr. Pargament is Professor, Department of Psychology, Bowling Green State University, Bowling Green, OH. (Address correspondence to Dr. Jenkins, Henry M. Jackson Foundation, 1 Taft Court, Suite 250, Rockville, MD 20850.) The opinions and assertions contained in this article are those of the authors and do not necessarily reflect those of the Uniformed Services University of the Health Sciences, the Henry M. Jackson Foundation for the Advancement of Military Medicine, or the United States Department of Defense.

[Haworth co-indexing entry note]: "Religion and Spirituality as Resources for Coping with Cancer." Jenkins, Richard A., and Kenneth I. Pargament. Co-published simultaneously in the *Journal of Psychosocial Oncology* (The Haworth Medical Press, an imprint of The Haworth Press, Inc.) Vol. 13, No. 1/2, 1995, pp. 51-74; and: *Psychosocial Resource Variables in Cancer Studies: Conceptual and Measurement Issues* (ed: Barbara Curbow, and Mark R. Somerfield), The Haworth Medical Press, an imprint of The Haworth Press, Inc., 1995, pp. 51-74. *[Single or multiple copies of this article are available from The Haworth Document Delivery Service: 1-800-342-9678, 9:00 a.m. - 5:00 p.m. (EST)].*

Religion and spirituality have received attention in a variety of studies of coping and adjustment in cancer patients. Drawing conclusions from this literature for purposes of further research or development of interventions is difficult because of the lack of specificity in the measurement of these variables and the absence of explicit paradigms for considering their role in patients' lives. This situation is not unique to cancer; religion and spirituality are treated in the same manner in other health-related literature (Jenkins, 1991).

Typically, religion has been examined through variables such as average church attendance, religious denomination, or single-item scales along the lines of "How religious are you?" Efforts to assess religious or spiritual needs have tended to be vague, using general terms such as "unmet spiritual or existential needs," without details regarding the nature of those needs. Few studies have examined the use of specific religious or spiritual beliefs, religious practices, or situations in which religious or spiritual beliefs may be particularly salient. Also, little attention has been given to how religion fits with other coping variables and how it can be integrated into the psychosocial care of patients.

Outside the psychosocial literature, issues such as the religious meaning of cancer have often been treated in the theological literature; however, these issues are relatively inaccessible to clinicians and researchers because they tend to appear in theologically oriented journals and often require some grounding in biblical texts. Because of the relatively secular background of people who work in fields such as psychology (Beit-Hallahmi, 1992; Larson et al., 1986; Martin & Carlson, 1988; Sarason, 1993), one also might expect some basic philosophical resistance to using a theological perspective to deal with psychosocial issues in cancer.

This article focuses on religion and spirituality as resources for coping with cancer. Here, religion refers to organized systems of belief and practice such as those found in formal denominations (e.g., Catholic, Jewish, Protestant, Moslem, Buddhist) or recognized systems of theological ideas (e.g., Calvinistic, Protestant, Evangelical Christian). Spirituality is more difficult to define, but it can be viewed best as efforts to consider metaphysical or transcendent aspects of everyday life as they relate to forces, supernatural and otherwise, that exist outside of the person. Hence, spirituality encompasses religion as well as many beliefs and practices from outside the normally defined religious sphere (e.g., "new age" philosophies; belief in a "higher power," as in 12-step groups; folkloric beliefs that are separate from or ancillary to a formal religion such as belief in the "evil eye"). Spirituality also can be an alternative label for metaphysical experiences that is used by people who have negative views of organized religion. Because of the overlap between what is religion and what is spirituality, the two concepts will be treated as one unless there is some empirical, theological, or practical reason to do otherwise.

We begin with general considerations involved in the investigation of religion and spirituality: that is, tensions between the religious and spiritual world and the worlds of psychological research and practice. Then we provide a brief review of existing literature, followed by a discussion of a taxonomy for integrating religious and nonreligious aspects of coping with cancer. Finally, we discuss strategies for capturing religious and spiritual phenomena in research and clinical settings.

TENSIONS WITH PSYCHOSOCIAL RESEARCH AND PRACTICE

To understand how cancer patients use religion and spirituality, one must examine the ways in which these factors may be alien to researchers and clinicians, along with the resultant heuristics and biases. Most clinicians come from secular backgrounds and tend to be less religious than their clients (Beit-Hallahmi, 1992; Larson et al., 1986). Similarly, researchers are less likely to acknowledge a belief in an afterlife than is the general public (Gallup & Proctor, 1982). Furthermore, psychotherapeutic thinkers tend to dismiss religion as "superstition" (Sarason, 1993), and medicine has had a long history of antipathy toward religion (Levin & Vanderpool, 1992).

Secular practitioners may commit the kinds of fallacies evident in the research literature: i.e., they may assume that all religions are the same and that practices such as church attendance and prayer mean the same thing regardless of one's religious background. These assumptions go against relatively obvious differences in religious doctrine that may have implications for coping and general health care. For example, Ebaugh, Richman, and Chafetz (1984) found that coping activities in response to crisis were highly variable between different religious groups. In their study, Charismatic Catholics turned to their group for emotional support, whereas Bahais coped through interpretation of writings and Christian Scientists focused on positive thinking.

Although denominational concerns are important, one also must recognize that religious beliefs and practices can be divorced from formal ties to any religious organization. When Jenkins (1985) interviewed cancer patients about their coping, it was not unusual for patients to make comments such as the following: "You know, I haven't been to church in 25 years, but having cancer has made me think about whether this disease may have some kind of meaning in terms of my place on earth." Similarly, one must recognize that even when people are committed to a particular religious denomination, they may disregard specific areas of religious doctrine. For example, people from a Christian tradition may discount the inevitability or purpose of an afterlife.

Pargament et al. (1988) provided one illustration of the differences and complexities in approaches to coping with a single religious group. In a sample drawn from Protestant denominations, they identified three distinct religious ways of maintaining a sense of agency and control in coping: (1) "collaborative" religious coping, in which God was defined as a partner who shared responsibility with the individual for problem solving, (2) "deferring" coping, in which the individual delegated responsibility to God while passively waiting for the outcome, and (3) "self-directed" coping, in which individuals assumed that God had given them the skills and resources to solve problems for themselves. More recently, Pargament et al. (1990) also found a fourth approach to religious coping based on strivings for mastery through attempts to influence the will of God by praying for positive outcomes or pleading for a miracle. Thus, even within a single religious tradition, simple utterances about God's will may have different meanings. What superficially appears to be fatalism may indeed be fatalistic; on the other hand, it may represent a more proactive, interactive attempt to maintain a sense of control in life.

Finally, researchers and clinicians may misunderstand religion and spirituality because they tend to classify religion as a passive way of coping (McCrae, 1984) or as a defense mechanism (Freud, 1961), precluding the possibility of proactive roles. Empirical studies do not lend much support to the stereotypical view of religion as a passive defense mechanism. In fact, several lines of evidence converge to suggest that at least some forms of religion are part of an active coping style: (1) factor analyses of general coping inventories generally have found that religious items fall into active rather than passive dimensions of coping (e.g., Folkman & Lazarus, 1988; Gil et al., 1989), (2) measures of religious commitment often relate to an internal rather than external locus of control (Jackson & Coursey, 1988; Shrauger & Silverman, 1971), and (3) some styles of religious coping have been associated with high levels of personal competence and initiative in problem solving (Carver, Scheier, & Weintraub, 1989; Pargament et al., 1988).

Despite the presence of evidence that supports religion as an active mode of coping, one must recognize that religion can be used in a variety of ways and thus defies easy categorization. For example, Dunkel-Schetter et al.'s factor analytic work (1992) suggests that some aspects of religion fall into passive coping factors (e.g., hoping for a miracle), whereas others load on more active coping factors (e.g., finding new faith). These authors also found that "religiosity" (a single-item measure of "strength of spiritual belief") relate to both cognitive reframing and behavioral escape-avoidance. Similarly, the coping styles delineated by Pargament et al. (1988), discussed earlier, illustrated how religion can fall outside of simple categories such as active and passive coping.

RELIGION AND ADAPTATION

Despite its limitations, the existing literature on religion and spirituality in cancer does provide a basis for understanding some of its importance to patients and can frame some useful hypotheses for the researcher, clinical practitioner, or both. Many cancer patients clearly view religion as personally salient, although figures have varied widely across studies (from 50 percent to 90 percent) (Jenkins & Pargament, 1988; Peteet, 1985-86; Spilka, Ladd, & David, 1993). Even among those who do not view religion as being highly important, religious activities such as prayer or consultation with clergy are common (Spilka, Ladd, & David, 1993). As many as one-third of all patients in some studies indicated that they had unmet spiritual or existential needs (e.g., Cella & Tross, 1986; Driever & McCorkle, 1984; Houts et al., 1986), which suggests that clinical care is often inattentive to this area of patients' lives.

A number of studies have found significant relations between religiousness and measures of adjustment, symptom management, or both. The presence of strong religious beliefs has been related to decreased levels of pain, anxiety, hostility, and social isolation as well as higher levels of life satisfaction in cancer patients (Acklin, Brown, & Mauger, 1983; Gibbs & Achterberg-Lawlis, 1978; Kaczorowski, 1989; Yates et al., 1981). Related concepts such as hope (Parsons, 1977), optimism, and freedom from regret (Weisman & Worden, 1976-77) also have been tied to better adjustment, as has church attendance (Acklin, Brown, & Mauger, 1983; Yates et al., 1981). In addition, religious or spiritual variables may be related to lower mortality rates among cancer patients (Gottschalk, 1974; Levin & Schiller, 1987). On the other hand, studies have suggested negative impacts on adjustment from religious variables such as frequent church attendance (Weisman, 1976) and fatalistic religious beliefs (Baider & Sarell, 1983). In general, these findings need to be viewed as suggestive rather than definitive because most studies have used highly simplistic measures of religion and have tested them through bivariate analyses (e.g., zero-order correlations or *t*-tests) rather than in highly elaborated multivariate models.

Mechanisms of Adaptation

One potential inference from existing research is that religion may facilitate coping in some patients and impede it in others. Perhaps differences in findings reflect situational factors or the impact of specific religious functions, beliefs, and practices. Because the role and scope of religion in these studies typically have been defined in a vague or general way, one also must extrapolate from work done in other populations or must examine descriptive works that have attempted to delineate roles and functions for religion and spirituality but have not related them directly to adjustment. Taken together, existing work on religion and cancer, along with more general research on religion and adjustment, can be organized into a taxonomy in which relations between religious resources, religious coping, and adjustment can be explored (see Figure 1).

This taxonomy illustrates how religious coping may serve different purposes and may be influenced by factors both religious and nonreligious in origin. Hence, background, situational, or resource variables may exert effects on adjustment through the religious coping processes and associated functions that they influence. These different classes of variables also may exert direct effects on self-management strategies and on adjustment; however, these pathways fall outside the topic of religious or spiritual coping and will not be discussed here. Many religious pathways to adjustment can be traced to ways that religion has been considered in general models of psychosocial functioning such as tension reduction (Freud, 1961), social integration and intimacy (Durkheim, 1951), meaning (Geertz, 1966), personal efficacy, and growth (Fromm, 1950). Because these models tap different, though often overlapping, religious functions, part of the strength of religion lies in its ability to serve multiple purposes. Therein also lies the complexity of religion. As we discussed earlier, clinicians and social/behavioral scientists often reduce religion to stereotypes, if they consider its role at all. Thus, they may ignore its value as an independent source of motivation.

Situational factors. Religious functions and activities may depend, in part, on the context of cancer in a particular person's life. Research with other populations suggests that religious coping tends to be used under conditions of serious personal threat such as a life-threatening illness more often than in other types of life events (Lindenthal et al., 1970; Pargament & Sullivan, 1981; Spilka & Schmidt, 1983). Under this rubric, one might assume that religion is more salient to coping when a cancer diagnosis is first made or at relapse (when the threat of cancer is arguably strongest), particularly given the compromise of patient adjustment associated with these events (e.g., Derogatis et al., 1983; Psychological Aspects of Breast Cancer Study Group, 1987; Silberfarb, Maurer, & Crouthamel, 1980; Weisman & Worden, 1976-77). Religion and spirituality might be considered in conjunction with factors that raise threats to

FIGURE 1. The Relations Between Religious Resources, Religious Coping, Nonreligious Factors, and Adjustment in Cancer Patients.

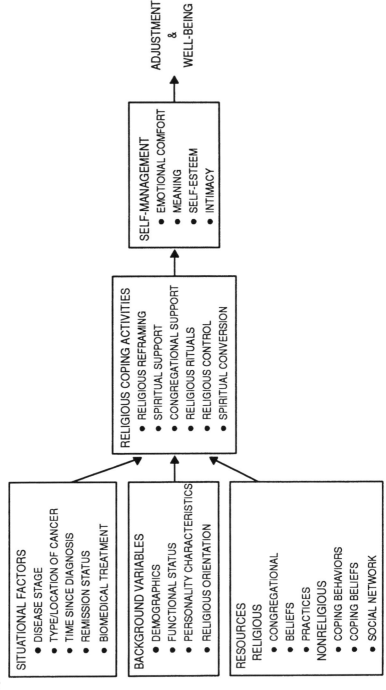

mortality, such as severe or relatively advanced disease. Such factors often compromise adjustment and well-being (Vinokur et al., 1989). Religious issues also may be important with respect to specific types or sites of a malignancy. Cancers that pose threats to self-image (e.g., when treatment involves disfiguring surgery) or important areas of personal functioning such as sexuality may have particular existential importance and stimulate the use of religious resources. Indeed, some research with these cancers has suggested that this may be the case (e.g., Cella & Tross, 1986). Finally, biomedical treatment may be important to the extent that some cancer treatments, such as allogeneic bone marrow transplantation, have serious mortality rates, and, in some cases, treatment may lengthen life without enhancing quality of life. Consequently, concerns about mortality and other issues that are salient to religious coping may vary as a function of medical intervention.

Background variables. Interacting with cancer-related situational factors may be fixed characteristics of a person or dispositional factors that remain relatively stable across situations. For example, demographic variables have shown some relation to religious coping in other populations. Some also have demonstrated specific effects on cancer-related adjustment. In the general population, religious coping appears to be used more often by women than men, African-Americans than Caucasians, older people than young adults, and adults with low socioeconomic status than adults with high socioeconomic status (e.g., Gurin, Veroff, & Feld, 1960; Mickley & Soeken, 1993; Spilka, Hood, & Gorsuch, 1985). Some demographic factors such as age affect the adjustment of people with cancer: Younger patients report more problems than do older patients (e.g., Vinokur et al., 1989). Functional status, which may or may not reflect impacts from cancer, needs consideration as well. Variables such as church attendance may not be useful in studying frail elderly individuals or people who are nonambulatory because of medical treatments (Levin, 1988).

Some background variables have more obvious or direct relevance to religious coping. If one is dealing with an unchurched population, contact with clergy may not be useful, whereas inspirational reading or prayer may be extremely important. Similarly, religious practices may vary if one is dealing with people from different religious backgrounds, especially if one or more religious groups are highly devotional or have distinct beliefs or practices (see, for example, Baider and Sarell's comparison, 1983, of Israeli women with breast cancer who were from secular European and religious "Oriental" backgrounds).

A widely studied background factor is religious orientation, a personality concept that has been influential in the general literature on psychology and religion. The paradigm of intrinsic versus extrinsic religious orientation (Allport, 1960) has been used to examine the role of religion in many contexts, including cancer. Intrinsic religion, according to Allport, reflects a deep commitment to one's faith and toward spiritual goals as well as the profound integration of religious beliefs and practices in life. If the intrinsically oriented live their religion, Allport said, the extrinsically oriented use their religion. This latter approach to religion is lightly held–a peripheral part of life to be used for personal and social rather than spiritual ends. Hence, an extrinsic orientation is essentially utilitarian and emphasizes religion for purposes of reinforcing social status, justifying one's way of life, or gaining a sense of safety.

Although extrinsic religiousness has failed to yield significant relations to coping and adjustment among cancer patients (Acklin, Brown, & Mauger, 1983; Gibbs & Achterberg-Lawlis, 1978; Johnson & Spilka, 1988; Mickley, Soeken, & Belcher, 1992), measures of intrinsic religiousness have been tied to higher levels of hope (Mickley, Soeken, & Belcher, 1992), perceptions of greater help through prayer and clergy visits (Johnson & Spilka, 1988), and lower levels of anger and hostility (Acklin, Brown, & Mauger, 1983). Gibbs and Achterberg-Lawlis (1978) found no relation between intrinsic religiousness and fear of death or physical discomfort among terminally ill cancer patients; however, studies outside of the cancer arena have found intrinsic religiousness to be negatively related to death anxiety (Kahoe & Dunn, 1975; Thorson & Powell, 1990).

Despite the presence of these significant findings, religious orientations have important theoretical and clinical limitations. Specifically, they do not address the concrete ways that religion is expressed in particular life situations. Intrinsic individuals may be deeply committed to a religious faith, but what meaning does this commitment have for understanding cancer, the solution of concrete problems, or how they sustain themselves emotionally? Conversely, both the intrinsically oriented person who seeks faith from religion and the extrinsic individual who sees church as a place for making respectable social contacts may have similar sources of religious coping (e.g., clergy and fellow congregants).

Pargament et al. (1990, 1992) have provided evidence that the specific religious coping activities one uses in critical life situations may mediate relations between general religious orientations and the outcomes of these life situations. Working with a sample of mainstream Christians, they found that religious orientation was associated with distinctive types of religious coping activities; however, these activities were more powerful predictors of the outcomes of negative events than were the religious orientations. This suggests the potential value of examining situation-specific religious coping efforts as they relate to the threats and challenges of cancer even if religious orientation also is investigated.

Beyond religious orientation, additional personality factors may influence religious coping directly or be important as general correlates of adjustment. For example, characteristic patterns of emotional control have been widely studied (e.g., Watson et al., 1984; Weisman & Worden, 1976-77); however, they have yielded conflicting outcomes with regard to adjustment.

Resource variables. Resource variables here refer to factors that are mobilized to deal with threats to one's adjustment and well-being. These may overlap to an extent with background variables such as personality factors (e.g., religious orientation). However, to the extent that personality variables tend to be relatively fixed and have limited predictive validity for specific situations (Mischel, 1968), they are not considered to be resources here. Instead, resources refer to what the lay person would see as "sources of help" or "things to fall back on." Resources can be viewed as the bases from which efforts to deal with stressful situations emerge. The identification of resources logically leads to specific coping activities and the self-management functions they exert to effect adjustment. Because both religious and nonreligious resources may be related to the enactment of religious coping activities, both resources are considered in the following paragraphs.

People may turn to a variety of religious resources in times of stress, including clergy and members of their congregation, if they are affiliated with a church or another place of worship. They may draw on general beliefs or practices and apply them to a specific situation (e.g., bargaining with God for more time, praying for a miraculous recovery).

Nonreligious sources of help in people's lives can affect religious coping. Tendencies toward specific types of coping behaviors may lead one to find ways to incorporate religion in an effort to maintain adjustment. Thoits (1986) suggested that if one coping strategy may help in a particular situation, then a similar social support strategy also may help. One can extend this logic to suggest that the efficacy of general coping strategies also may predict the efficacy, and perhaps the likelihood, of using an analogous religious coping strategy. Hence, if one seeks to cope with the uncertainty of cancer by finding meaning in the experience, religion may be a part of this search (Taylor, Lichtman, & Wood, 1984). Similarly, if one seeks to reframe the situation posed by mortality in more positive terms, religion may be applied in this way (e.g., McIntosh, Silver, & Wortman, 1993). These kinds of relations between analogous religious and nonreligious coping activities have been obtained in noncancer populations (Pargament et al., 1990). Beliefs may operate in a manner similar to coping behavior. For example, beliefs that control over cancer exists outside the person may motivate efforts to seek control through interchange with God (Jenkins & Pargament, 1988).

On the other hand, the inadequacy of personal resources may lead one toward religious coping. Appraisal of a situation as a loss is associated with greater use of religious coping (McCrae, 1984), as is dealing with situations that are poorly explained in objective, "scientific" terms (e.g., Spilka & Schmidt, 1983).

Religious Coping, Self-Management, and Adjustment

Once the paths to religious coping have been delineated, discussing the functions it serves in self-management and how these functions affect adjustment is important. Descriptive studies of cancer patients have indicated that religion is often viewed as a source of comfort, solace, and support (Castles & Keith, 1979; Kesselring et al., 1986; Spilka, Spangler, & Nelson, 1983), findings that have occurred in other populations as well (e.g., Fichter, 1981; O'Brien, 1982; Wright, Pratt, & Schmall, 1985). Spilka, Ladd, and David (1993) found that prayer helped breast cancer patients reduce their fears and manage their emotions. Studies also suggest that religion may be used to explain the etiology of cancer or one's response to its treatment and, more generally, to find meaning in the illness (e.g., "it's God's will") (Gotay, 1985; Linn, Linn, & Stein, 1982; Taylor, Lichtman, & Wood, 1984). At least one study has suggested that cancer patients who have strong religious beliefs are more likely to use cognitive reframing (e.g., to focus on the positive) as a coping technique, although no data were presented regarding whether religious cognitions were involved (Dunkel-Schetter et al., 1992).

Research with other populations has suggested that religion can be used to reframe problems in a positive way (Wright, Pratt, & Schmall, 1985) and to use this positive reframing to maintain or regain emotional homeostasis (Newman & Pargament, 1987). Religious systems of beliefs have been shown to help a person sustain a sense of justice and benevolence in ostensibly unfair situations such as those in which bad things seem to be happening to good people (e.g., lung cancer in a nonsmoker) (Pargament & Hahn, 1986). This sustenance appears to be based on (1) faith in each person's unique spiritual destiny, (2) the proposition that no person will be given more than he or she can handle, and (3) the notion that misfortune provides special opportunities for spiritual growth. Religious coping also enhances perceived control, builds self-esteem (Spilka, Shaver, & Kirkpatrick, 1985), and provides emotional release and intimacy, as in the case of religious services (Griffith, Young, & Smith, 1984). In addition, many coping functions of prayer have been noted: for example, requests for guidance or intervention from God, desires for growth, or feelings of closeness to God (Clark, 1958).

RELIGION AND SPIRITUALITY IN RESEARCH

The taxonomy described here illustrates some of the religious variables that can be useful to collect, given particular kinds of situations. As such, they provide a means of overcoming the vague approach taken in the past. The multiple roles and settings for religion in coping suggest the need to consider practical issues in relation to collecting data on such a complex subject. Practice settings such as clinics and hospitals typically require that clinical care take precedence over research, except when the two are inextricably linked (i.e., experimental treatment protocols). Furthermore, gatekeepers in research settings (e.g., physicians, nurses, administrators) may make access to patients contingent upon receiving "practical feedback" from the research data. This can constrain the range of research topics covered and may make religious or spiritual variables seem esoteric compared to issues such as neuropsychiatric functioning or self-care capabilities. These circumstances create a reliance on brief self-report questionnaires when, unfortunately, few such measures have been devised to study religious and spiritual coping variables.

Existing Instruments

Box 1 outlines items from the few instruments that have been developed to capture religious and spiritual coping. Among these, Maton (1989) developed a brief (three-item) measure of spiritual support that was predictive of less depression and greater self-esteem in three highly stressed groups. Carver, Scheier, and Weintraub (1989) derived a four-item Turning to Religion coping subscale from factor analysis of their multidimensional COPE measure of general coping. This subscale was positively associated with measures of optimism and information seeking under stress. Pargament et al. (1988) published short forms (six items each) of the three styles of religious coping that were discussed earlier. Additional studies with various populations have tied these three styles to different levels of psychosocial competence, physical health (McIntosh & Spilka, 1990), and psychological adjustment (Schaefer & Gorsuch, 1991). Pargament et al. (1990) also published a more extensive set of six factor analytically derived subscales regarding religious coping activities that could be used selectively in further research (see Box 1). These subscales have demonstrated an ability to predict adjustment to significant negative events beyond the effects of nonreligious measures.

Significantly, all the measures noted here have been used to determine how religious and spiritual coping may be related to

BOX 1. Illustrative Items from Religious Coping Scales.

Spiritual support (Maton, 1989)
I experience God's love and caring on a regular basis.
Religious faith has not been central to my coping.

Turning to religion (Carver, Sheier, & Weintraub, 1989)
I seek God's help.
I put my trust in God.

Three styles of religious coping (Pargament et al., 1988)
Collaborative style
  When it comes to deciding how to solve a problem, God and I work
    together as partners.
  When I feel nervous or anxious about a problem, I work with God to
    find a way to relieve my worries.
Deferring style
  I do not think about different solutions to my problems because God
    provides them for me.
  When a situation makes me nervous, I wait for God to take those
    feelings away.
Self-directing style
  I act to solve my problems without God's help.
  After I've gone through a rough time, I try to make sense of it
    without relying on God.

Religious coping activities (Pargament et al., 1990)
Spiritually based coping
  I realized that God was trying to strengthen me.
  I trusted that God would not let anything terrible happen to me.
Religious good deeds
  I confessed my sins.
  I provided help to other church members.
Religious discontent
  I felt angry with or distant from God.
  I questioned my religious beliefs and faith.
Religious support
  I received support from clergy.
  I received support from other members of the church.
Pleading
  I asked for a miracle.
  I bargained with God to make things better.
Religious avoidance
  I focused on the world-to-come rather than the problems of this world.
  I prayed or read the Bible to keep my mind off of my problems.

other aspects of coping (e.g., social support, perceived control). Consequently, they illustrate the importance of integrating religious and spiritual coping into a larger theoretical framework rather than viewing it as an isolated area of study, which typically occurs with measures such as church attendance.

Development of New Measures

The limited number of measures that address religious and spiritual coping and the current state of the literature create a situation in which one may wish to develop new measures or find ways to elaborate on existing ones. These situations can be addressed through a number of research strategies, including both qualitative and quantitative approaches. Often, qualitative and quantitative studies pose "either or" alternatives rather than complementary approaches (see, for example, Tebes & Kraemer, 1991). However, qualitative strategies such as case studies and focus groups can be extremely valuable in exploring concepts and processes that are poorly understood and not easily placed into an objective questionnaire format. As such, they can serve as a step toward developing quantitative measures (Zeller, 1993). Similar methods also are helpful in translating largely hypothetical, quantitatively measured constructs (e.g., perceived control, social support) into specific, concrete intervention targets in patients' daily lives.

One illustration of the tandem use of quantitative and qualitative techniques comes from the first author's doctoral dissertation, a study of patient coping. This study examined perceived control over cancer–quantitatively through scales and qualitatively through open-ended questions about how various forces (self, powerful others, chance, and God) exercised control–as a follow-up to the scales. This strategy made it possible to see an interplay between sources of control (e.g., God working through physicians, gaining access to God's power through prayer) that would not have been obvious from an analysis of the quantitative data. Although many people did not identify strongly with organized religion, this process also made it evident that religion was given universal importance (Jenkins, 1985). This strategy was time-consuming; however, other investigators might use open-ended written questions in much the same way, particularly in a relatively well-educated population.

Another illustration comes from Pargament et al.'s use (1988, 1990) of intensive case study interviews in developing scales to measure religious coping styles and the use of specific religious coping activities. Interviews probed how respondents used religion in their daily lives and how they applied it to recent significant problems. This approach permitted assessment of ways in which religious or spiritual coping was part of more general coping processes, which helped to clarify the relations between religious or spiritual coping and processes such as perceived control, social support, mastery, reframing, and derivation of meaning. Although case study interviews require relatively few subjects, different segments of the population of interest must be sampled adequately and the nonrepresentative nature of the most cooperative and articulate interview participants must be recognized.

A third illustration comes from the first author's use (Jenkins, in preparation) of focus groups to explore religious or spiritual issues with people infected with HIV and to adapt to this population religious coping measures previously developed by the second author and colleagues. Although many members were not active in a church and some felt estranged from organized religion, feedback from the groups indicated that religion was an important factor in coping with HIV and that religious or spiritual beliefs and practices were relevant. Like case study interviews, focus groups may have limited usefulness because of their representativeness, and, again, one must be certain that relevant segments of the population of interest are sampled to some degree. In addition, group dynamics may influence the discourse and behavior of group members (Zeller, 1993). One of our focus groups was dominated by an especially vocal, self-described nonreligious person who saw little value in probing the subject of religious coping. Other viewpoints were not expressed assertively, and the representativeness of this person's views was difficult to gauge.

RELIGION AND SPIRITUALITY IN CLINICAL PRACTICE

Despite the tensions between religion, spirituality, and the mental health professions noted previously, some authors have attempted to reconcile religion and mental health practice, at least at a general level and in some specific contexts such as bereavement. Miller (1985) noted that therapeutic strategies may result in more lasting behavioral change if they reflect core beliefs or values. Furthermore, Bergin (1985) observed that therapeutic efforts are inherently value-laden and make many assumptions about optimal patterns of behavior (e.g., personal responsibility and autonomy, self-awareness, interpersonal commitment, and possession of a mature value system), which are easily translated into religious or spiritual systems and, indeed, permeate diverse Judeo-Christian traditions. In this respect, the clinician's task is to determine whether religious or spiritual systems of thought that are relevant to therapeutic values can be used as a vehicle for facilitating behavioral change in the same ways that other aspects of one's phenomenology are addressed in common therapeutic approaches. Particularly for the secular clinician, this means going beyond stereotyped notions of religion and what constitutes a religious patient.

Just as the researcher must go beyond the temptation to use a "quick and dirty" scale to study religious coping, clinicians must go beyond simple questions that may not encompass a patient's religious experience. Hence, asking if someone is religious, attends church, and so forth may be less important than asking how that person views the religious or spiritual significance of the events in his or her life and how religion may be part of the healing process. In times of crisis, religion may be expressed through traditional beliefs and practices; however, it may take other forms such as quasireligious practices such as yoga, meditation, or visualization. It can involve life-style changes with religious or moral components such as becoming more attentive to the needs of others or attempting to find meaning and significance in everyday events. Sometimes the parallels to religious belief or practice may not be obvious to patients or clinicians. Patients may seek to let go of pain or suffering by restructuring their lives around certain values or commitments, a process not unlike Buddhism. However, patients may not think of this as a religious practice; indeed, the thought of adopting an Asian religion may seem odd to them. Yet the notion that this source of action has a religious or quasireligious precedent may help in understanding how to make changes.

The clinician must be willing to learn more about the world's religions in general and the patient's religious world in particular. This is a tall order–one that many clinicians may lack the time or inclination to pursue. Major problems can be avoided, however, if the clinician remembers a few key points. First, religion and spirituality can serve many purposes (e.g., support, solace, personal meaning) that express themselves in many different ways under stressful circumstances. Second, even seemingly unusual beliefs or practices may have a role in coping (e.g., seeking solace in the reading of sacred texts). Third, whether the religious dimension is part of the problem or part of the solution may depend, not only on the particular beliefs and practices that are manifested, but also on the "fit" of religion to the specific challenges patients face, the resources and burdens they bring to coping, and their aspirations in life. In these respects, religion may not become important to a patient's coping until some ambiguity occurs with respect to the efficacy of the treatment or concerns are raised about his or her mortality. Finally, clinicians can seek out sources of religious expertise as consultants and collaborators. Traditionally, relations between the worlds of religion and mental health have been one sided, with clergy making far more referrals to mental health professionals than they receive in return (Carson, 1976; Meylink & Gorsuch, 1986). Yet, as the study of religion, illness, and coping expands, the fact that mental health professionals also have much to learn from and about religion in times of crisis becomes clear.

REFERENCES

Acklin, M. W., Brown, E. C., & Mauger, P. A. (1983). The role of religious values in coping with cancer. *Journal of Health & Religion, 22*, 322-333.

Allport, G. W. (1960). *The individual and his religion.* New York: Macmillan.

Baider, L., & Sarell, M. (1983). Perceptions and causal attributions of Israeli women with breast cancer concerning their illness: The effects of ethnicity and religiosity. *Psychotherapy & Psychosomatics, 39*, 136-143.

Beit-Hallahmi, B. (1992). *Prolegomena to the psychological study of religion.* Lewisburg, PA: Bucknell University Press.

Bergin, A. E. (1985). Proposed values for guiding and evaluating counseling and psychotherapy. *Counseling & Values, 29*, 99-116.

Carson, R. J. (1976). *Mental health centers and local clergy: A sourcebook of sample projects.* Washington, DC: Community Mental Health Institute.

Carver, C. S., Scheier, M. F., & Weintraub, J. K. (1989). Assessing coping strategies: A theoretically-based approach. *Journal of Personality & Social Psychology,* *56,* 267-283.

Castles, M. R., & Keith, P. M. (1979). Patient concerns, emotional resources, and perceptions of patient and nurse roles. *Omega: Journal of Death & Dying, 10,* 27-33.

Cella, D. F., & Tross, S. (1986). Psychological adjustment to survival from Hodgkin's disease. *Journal of Consulting & Clinical Psychology, 54,* 616-622.

Clark, W. (1958). *The psychology of religion.* New York: Macmillan.

Derogatis, L. R., Morrow, G. R., Fetting, J., Penman, D., Piasetsky, S., Schmale, A. M., Henrichs, M., & Carnicke, C. L. M. (1983). The prevalence of psychiatric disorders among cancer patients. *Journal of the American Medical Association, 249,* 751-757.

Driever, M. J., & McCorkle, R. (1984). Patient concerns at 3 and 6 months post diagnosis. *Cancer Nursing, 7,* 235-241.

Dunkel-Schetter, C., Feinstein, L. G., Taylor, S. E., & Falke, R. L. (1992). Patterns of coping with cancer. *Health Psychology, 11,* 79-87.

Durkheim, E. (1951). *Suicide.* New York: Free Press.

Ebaugh, H., Richman, K., & Chafetz, J. (1984). Life crises among the religiously committed: Do sectarian differences matter? *Journal for the Scientific Study of Religion, 23,* 19-31.

Fichter, J. H. (1981). *Religion and pain: The spiritual dimensions of health care.* New York: Crossroads.

Folkman, S., & Lazarus, R. S. (1988). Coping as a mediator of emotion. *Journal of Personality & Social Psychology, 54,* 466-475.

Freud, S. (1961). *The future of an illusion* (1927). New York: W. W. Norton.

Fromm, E. (1950). *Psychoanalysis and religion.* New Haven: Yale University Press.

Gallup, G., & Proctor, W. (1982). *Adventures in immortality.* New York: McGraw-Hill.

Geertz, C. (1966). Religion as a cultural system. In M. Banton (Ed.), *Anthropological approaches to the study of religion* (pp. 1-46). London, England: Tavistock.

Gibbs, H. W., & Achterberg-Lawlis, J. (1978). Spiritual values and death anxiety: Implications for counseling with terminal cancer patients. *Journal of Counseling Psychology, 25,* 563-569.

Gil, K. M., Abrams, M. R., Phillips, G., & Keefe, F. J. (1989). Sickle-cell disease pain: Relation of coping strategies to adjustment. *Journal of Consulting & Clinical Psychology, 57,* 725-731.

Gotay, C. C. (1985). Why me? Attributions and adjustment by cancer patients and their mates at two stages in the disease process. *Social Science & Medicine, 20,* 825-831.

Gottschalk, L. A. (1974). A hope scale applicable to verbal samples. *Archives of General Psychiatry, 30,* 779-785.

Griffith, E., Young, J., & Smith, D. (1984). An analysis of the therapeutic elements in a black church service. *Hospital & Community Psychiatry, 35,* 464-469.

Gurin, G., Veroff, J., & Feld, S. (1960). *Americans view their mental health: A nationwide interview survey.* New York: Basic Books.

Houts, P. S., Yasko, J. M., Kahn, S. B., Schlezel, G. W., & Marconi, K. M. (1986). Unmet psychological, social, and economic needs of persons with cancer in Pennsylvania. *Cancer, 58,* 2355-2361.

Jackson, L. E., & Coursey, R. D. (1988). The relationship of God control and internal locus of control to intrinsic religious motivation, coping, and purpose in life. *Journal for the Scientific Study of Religion, 27,* 399-410.

Jenkins, R. A. (1985). An investigation of cognitive attributes of coping in medical patients. Unpublished doctoral dissertation, Bowling Green State University, Bowling Green, OH.

Jenkins, R. A. (1991). Toward a psychosocial conceptualization of religion as a resource in cancer care and prevention. *Prevention in Human Services, 10,* 91-105.

Jenkins, R. A. (In preparation). Religion and HIV: Implications for research and intervention. *Journal of Social Issues.*

Jenkins, R. A., & Pargament, K. I. (1988). Cognitive appraisals and psychological adjustment in cancer patients. *Social Science & Medicine, 23,* 186-196.

Johnson, S. C., & Spilka, B. (1988, November). Coping with breast cancer: The role of religion. Paper presented at the annual meeting of the Society of the Scientific Study of Religion, Chicago, IL.

Kaczorowski, J. M. (1989). Spiritual well-being and anxiety in adults diagnosed with cancer. *Hospice Journal, 5,* 105-116.

Kahoe, R. D., & Dunn, R. F. (1975). The fear of death and religious attitudes and behavior. *Journal for the Scientific Study of Religion, 14,* 379-382.

Kesselring, A., Dodd, M. J., Lindsey, A. M., & Strauss, A. L. (1986). Attitudes of patients living in Switzerland about cancer and its treatment. *Cancer Nursing, 9,* 77-85.

Larson, D. B., Pattison, E. M., Blazer, D. G., Omran, A. R., & Kaplan, B. H. (1986). Systematic analysis of research on religious variables in four major psychiatric journals. *American Journal of Psychiatry, 143,* 329-334.

Levin, J. S. (1988). Religious factors in aging, adjustment, and health: A theoretical overview. *Journal of Religion & Aging, 4,* 133-146.

Levin, J. S., & Schiller, P. L. (1987). Is there a religious factor in health? *Journal of Religion & Health, 26,* 9-36.

Levin, J. S., & Vanderpool, H. Y. (1992). Religious factors in physical health and the prevention of illness. In K. I. Pargament, K. I. Maton, & R. E. Hess (Eds.), *Religion and prevention in mental health: Research, vision, and action* (pp. 83-104). New York: The Haworth Press, Inc.

Lindenthal, J. J., Myers, J. K., Pepper, M. P., & Stein, M. S. (1970). Mental status and religious behavior. *Journal for the Scientific Study of Religion, 9,* 143-149.

Linn, M. W., Linn, B. S., & Stein, S. R. (1982). Beliefs about causes of cancer in cancer patients. *Social Science & Medicine, 16,* 835-839.

Martin, J. E., & Carlson, C. R. (1988). Spiritual dimensions of health psychology. In W. R. Miller & Martin (Eds.), *Behavior therapy and religion: Integrating spiritual and behavioral approaches to change.* Newbury Park, CA: Sage Publications.

Maton, K. I. (1989). The stress-buffering role of spiritual support: Cross-sectional and prospective investigations. *Journal for the Scientific Study of Religion, 28,* 310-323.

McCrae, R. R. (1984). Situational determinants of coping response: Loss, threat, and challenge. *Journal of Personality & Social Psychology, 46,* 919-928.

McIntosh, D., & Spilka, B. (1990). Religion and physical health: The role of personal faith and control. In M. G. Lynn & D. O. Moberg (Eds.), *Research in the social scientific study of religion* (Vol. 2, pp. 167-194). Greenwich, CT: JAI Press.

McIntosh, D. N., Silver, R. C., & Wortman, C. B. (1993). Religion's role in adjustment to a negative life event: Coping with the loss of a child. *Journal of Personality & Social Psychology, 65,* 812-821.

Meylink, W. D., & Gorsuch, R. L. (1986). New perspectives for clergy-psychologist referrals. *Journal of Psychology & Christianity, 5,* 62-70.

Mickley, J., & Soeken, K. (1993). Religiousness and hope in Hispanic and Anglo-American women with breast cancer. *Oncology Nursing Forum, 20,* 1171-1177.

Mickley, J. R., Soeken, K., & Belcher, A. (1992). Spiritual well-being, religiousness, and hope among women with breast cancer. *IMAGE: Journal of Nursing Scholarship, 24,* 267-272.

Miller, W. R. (1985). Motivation for treatment: A review. *Psychological Bulletin, 98,* 84-107.

Mischel, W. (1968). *Personality and assessment.* New York: John Wiley & Sons.

Newman, J., & Pargament, K. (1987, November). The role of religion in the problem solving process. Paper presented at the annual meeting of the Society for the Scientific Study of Religion, Louisville, KY.

O'Brien, M. E. (1982). Religious faith and adjustment to long-term hemodialysis. *Journal of Religion & Health, 21,* 68-80.

Pargament, K. I., & Hahn, J. (1986). God and the just world: Causal and coping attributions to God in health situations. *Journal for the Scientific Study of Religion, 25,* 193-207.

Pargament, K. K., & Sullivan, M. S. (1981). Examining attributions of control across diverse personal situations: A psychosocial perspective. Paper presented at the annual meeting of the American Psychological Association, Los Angeles, CA.

Pargament, K., Grevengoed, N., Hathaway, W., Kennell, J., Newman, J., & Jones, W. (1988). Religion and problem solving: Three styles of coping. *Journal for the Scientific Study of Religion, 27,* 90-104.

Pargament, K. I., Ensing, D. S., Falgout, K., Olsen, H., Reilly, B., Van Haitsma, K., & Warren, R. (1990). God help me: (I) Religious coping efforts as predictors of the outcomes to significant negative life events. *American Journal of Community Psychology, 18*, 793-824.

Pargament, K., Olsen, H., Reilly, B., Falgout, K., Ensing, D., & Van Haitsma, K. (1992). God help me: (II) The relationship of religious orientations to religious coping with negative life events. *Journal for the Scientific Study of Religion, 31*, 504-513.

Parsons, J. B. (1977). A descriptive study of intermediate stage terminally ill cancer patients at home. *Nursing Digest, 5*, 1-26.

Peteet, J. R. (1985-86). Religious issues presented by cancer patients seen in psychiatric consultation. *Journal of Psychosocial Oncology, 3*(1), 53-66.

Psychological Aspects of Breast Cancer Study Group. (1987). Psychological response to mastectomy: A prospective comparison study. *Cancer, 59*, 189-196.

Sarason, S. B. (1993). American psychology, and the needs for transcendence and community. *American Journal of Community Psychology, 21*, 185-202.

Schaefer, C. A., & Gorsuch, R. L. (1991). Psychological adjustment and religiousness: The multivariate belief-motivation theory of religiousness. *Journal for the Scientific Study of Religion, 30*, 448-461.

Shrauger, J. S., & Silverman, R. E. (1971). The relationship of religious background and participation to locus of control. *Journal for the Scientific Study of Religion, 10*, 11-16.

Silberfarb, P. M., Maurer, L. H., & Crouthamel, C. S. (1980). Psychosocial aspects of neoplastic disease: I. Functional status of breast cancer patients during different treatment regimens. *American Journal of Psychiatry, 137*, 450-455.

Spilka, B., & Schmidt, G. (1983). General attribution theory for the psychology of religion: The influence of event-character on attributions to God. *Journal for the Scientific Study of Religion, 22*, 326-329.

Spilka, B., Hood, R. W., & Gorsuch, R. L. (1985). *The psychology of religion: An empirical approach.* Englewood Cliffs, NJ: Prentice-Hall.

Spilka, B., Ladd, K., & David, J. (1993). Religion and coping with breast cancer: Possible roles for prayer and form of personal faith (Technical Report). Atlanta, GA: American Cancer Society.

Spilka, B., Shaver, P., & Kirkpatrick, L. (1985). A general attribution theory for the psychology of religion. *Journal for the Scientific Study of Religion, 24*, 1-20.

Spilka, B., Spangler, J. D., & Nelson, C. B. (1983). Spiritual support in life threatening illness. *Journal of Religion & Health, 22*, 98-104.

Taylor, S. E., Lichtman, R. R., & Wood, J. V. (1984). Attributions, beliefs about control, and adjustment to breast cancer. *Journal of Personality & Social Psychology, 46*, 489-502.

Tebes, J. K., & Kraemer, D. T. (1991). Quantitative and qualitative knowing in mutual support research: Some lessons from the recent history of scientific psychology. *American Journal of Community Psychology, 19*, 739-756.

Thoits, P. A. (1986). Social support as coping assistance. *Journal of Consulting & Clinical Psychology, 54*, 416-423.

Thorson, J. A., & Powell, F. C. (1990). Meanings of death and intrinsic religiosity. *Journal of Clinical Psychology, 46*, 379-391.

Vinokur, A. D., Threatt, B. A., Caplan, R. D., & Zimmerman, B. L. (1989). Physical and psychosocial functioning and adjustment to breast cancer: Long-term follow-up of a screening population. *Cancer, 63*, 394-405.

Watson, M., Greer, S., Blake, S., & Shrapnell, K. (1984). Reaction to a diagnosis of breast cancer: Relationship between denial, delay, and rates of psychological morbidity. *Cancer, 53*, 2008-2012.

Weisman, A. D. (1976). A model for psychosocial phasing in cancer. *General Hospital Psychiatry, 1*, 187-195.

Weisman, A. D., & Worden, J. W. (1976-77). The existential plight in cancer: Significance of the first 100 days. *International Journal of Psychiatry in Medicine, 7*, 1-15.

Wright, S., Pratt, C., & Schmall, V. (1985). Spiritual support for caregivers of dementia patients. *Journal of Religion & Health, 24*, 31-38.

Yates, J., Chalmer, B., St. James, P., Follansbee, M., & McKegney, F. (1981). Religion in patients with advanced cancer. *Medical & Pediatric Oncology, 9*, 121-128.

Zeller, R. A. (1993). Combining qualitative and quantitative techniques to develop culturally sensitive measures. In D. G. Ostrow & R. C. Kessler (Eds.), *Methodological issues in AIDS behavioral research* (pp. 96-116). New York: Plenum Press.

The Role of Social Support in Adaptation to Cancer and to Survival

Christina G. Blanchard, MSW, PhD
Terrance L. Albrecht, PhD
John C. Ruckdeschel, MD, FACP
Charles H. Grant III, MA
Rebecca Malcolm Hemmick, MA

SUMMARY. Social support continues to be studied by many investigators as a variable associated with adaptation to the stress of cancer and its treatment. Recent selected studies are reviewed and limitations of the studies are noted, including the predominance of cross-sectional designs, lack of agreement on instruments to use to assess social supports and outcome measures, and the dearth of substantive models for guiding research and interventions. Although studies have also explored the relationship between support and survival, results are inconclusive. Future studies should include longitudinal designs, analyze support as an interactional process based on mutual influence, and explore the relationship between social support and the domains of quality of life (in addition to mood). *[Article copies are available from The Haworth Document Delivery Service: 1-800-342-9678.]*

Dr. Blanchard is Professor of Medicine and Psychiatry, Division of Medical Oncology, Albany Medical College, A-52, Albany, NY 12208-3479. Dr. Albrecht is Professor, Department of Community & Family Health, University of South Florida, Tampa, FL. Dr. Ruckdeschel is Professor of Medicine and Center Director, H. Lee Moffitt Cancer Center and Research Institute, Tampa, FL. Mr. Grant and Ms. Hemmick are PhD candidates, Department of Communication, University of South Florida, Tampa.

[Haworth co-indexing entry note]: "The Role of Social Support in Adaptation to Cancer and to Survival." Blanchard, Christina G. et al. Co-published simultaneously in the *Journal of Psychosocial Oncology* (The Haworth Medical Press, an imprint of The Haworth Press, Inc.) Vol. 13, No. 1/2, 1995, pp. 75-95; and: *Psychosocial Resource Variables in Cancer Studies: Conceptual and Measurement Issues* (ed: Barbara Curbow, and Mark R. Somerfield), The Haworth Medical Press, an imprint of The Haworth Press, Inc., 1995, pp. 75-95. *[Single or multiple copies of this article are available from The Haworth Document Delivery Service: 1-800-342-9678, 9:00 a.m. - 5:00 p.m. (EST)].*

Social support continues to be widely studied as a factor that has an impact on the patient's adjustment to cancer and, more recently, as a potential mediator of survival. Since Wortman's comprehensive review of this topic in 1984 (updated by Broadhead and Kaplan in 1991), more than 300 studies attest to the saliency of this topic for researchers and clinicians. The purpose of this article is to provide a selected review of recent key studies, to synthesize the implications of this work for clinicians in oncology settings, and to propose areas of needed research.

DEFINITIONS AND OVERVIEW

Despite a lack of specificity in definitions and measures of support, reasonable consensus exists regarding the essential components of support. Cohen and Syme (1985) suggested that a distinction between structure and function is inherent in the most commonly used measures. Structure is generally measured by self-reports of ties to others, along which supportive resources can be expected to flow. Structural indexes that have been studied include role designation, size, density/integration, reciprocity, and homogeneity/heterogeneity of social support networks. (See Albrecht & Adelman, 1987, for a review of major structural properties for all levels of analysis of social support networks.) Function refers to the acts performed for a distressed individual by significant others, including family, friends, and health care professionals. These functions typically include instrumental aid, socioemotional aid, and informational aid (see Thoits, 1986). Instrumental aid refers to actions or materials provided by others that assist the individual in enacting normal role responsibilities. Socioemotional assistance refers to assertions or demonstrations of love, esteem, caring, or group belonging. Informational aid refers to communications of opinion or fact that are relevant to current stressors, such as advice or information that might make the individual's life situation less stressful.

The impact of social support on broad aspects of health and well-being has been of great interest. Support has been associated with such outcomes as reduced sorrow or distress, improved recovery from illness or trauma, and resolution of conflict. Social support has been associated with an increase in resistance to infection and disease, improvement in psychological adjustments and perceptions of self-efficacy and, potentially, reductions in mortality (see Albrecht, Burleson, & Goldsmith, 1994).

Support has been posited as having a buffering effect for cancer patients: that is, support protects the patient from the full onslaught of stressors produced by the disease experience when interpersonal resources are available and responsive to the patient's needs (Cohen & Wills, 1985). Drawing on Lazarus and Folkman's appraisal theory (1984), Thoits (1986) suggested that social support might be usefully reconceptualized as coping assistance, or the active participation of significant others in an individual's stress-management efforts (see, also, Nelles et al., 1991). The use of social support, like other coping strategies, would help the patient change the situation, the meaning of the situation, the emotional reaction to the situation, or all three. If successful, the problematic demands would be altered or eliminated and the anxiety or depression accompanying the demands would be managed better.

Matt and Dean (1993) questioned the assumption that there are causal effects of social support on distress. They hypothesized that distressed people might withdraw from interactions, causing potential sources of support to withdraw. Using structural equation modeling and a longitudinal design, they studied the complex relationship between friends' support and psychological distress among 749 elderly people and found that over a 22-month interval, low support from friends among the old-old (71 years and older) led to higher psychological distress and that high psychological distress led to less support from friends. This was not found for the young-old (50-70 years). Matt and Dean suggested a reciprocal causation: The old-old are particularly vulnerable to psychological distress when losing friends' support and are vulnerable to losing that support when experiencing psychological distress. Their study points to the need for continued investigation of the correlation between social support and outcome measures before causality can be assumed.

Albrecht and colleagues (Albrecht & Adelman, 1987, Burleson, Albrecht, & Sarason, 1994) have emphasized that for the past 20 years, scholars have focused on outcomes of supportive behaviors rather than on the nature of the process of communication in which support is provided. In contrast, Albrecht and Adelman (1987) postulated that social support is a communication process in which supporters and receivers mutually influence one another by reducing uncertainty and increasing a sense of personal control over their environments. They not only have discussed the benefits of support but also have explored the risks and costs of supportive communication for providers and recipients (see Albrecht, Burleson, & Goldsmith, 1994). For example, the risks and costs for recipients include embarrassment; fear of appearing weak or less competent; concerns about imposing, becoming overly dependent, being obligated; and anxiety over potential rejection. Providers can suffer a drainage of tangible resources; the stresses of obligation, frustration, or responsibility; and the fears of their own vulnerabilities and mortality.

Wortman and Dunkel-Schetter (1979, 1987) and Wortman (1984) suggested another theoretical approach. Cancer patients can be seen as victims of an uncontrollable event. Like all such victims, they are in need of special reassurance from others. This is particularly difficult for the cancer patient because the fears and stigma associated with the disease may lead significant others to avoid the patient, avoid communication about the cancer, or engage in forced cheerfulness. However, Zemore and Shepel (1989) found that women with breast cancer received greater emotional support from family and friends than did a group of women with benign breast lumps. They suggested that the victimization hypothesis might have been supported if patients were sicker, thus heightening the fears of others and resulting in increased avoidance. In contrast, Tempelaar et al. (1989) found that cancer patients who were more seriously ill reported receiving more help and support than did those who were less ill.

Dakof and Taylor (1990) suggested that the victimization hypothesis might apply more specifically to some relationships than to others. During interviews with 55 cancer patients, they found that this hypothesis applied more to interactions with friends and acquaintances than to interactions with close family members. They concluded that withdrawal or avoidance is more difficult for family members than for friends and acquaintances. However, their respondents did report more helpful than unhelpful actions from family, friends, and health care professionals. The source of support was important: Intimate others were valued more for emotional support, whereas physicians were valued more for informational support. Clearly, the recipient, the provider, and the interaction need to be studied to specify further the helpful and unhelpful types and sources of support and thus specify under what circumstances the victimization hypothesis may be correct.

REVIEW OF SELECTED LITERATURE

We reviewed the research literature from 1987-1993. The sample sizes, types and stages of cancer, instruments, and major findings in selected studies are summarized in Table 1.

Social Support and Psychosocial Adaptation

Probably the most important (and least ambiguous) finding is that patients who confide their fears and concerns to a loving and supportive spouse or close friend seem to fare better emotionally. For example, Dunkel-Schetter et al. (1992), using The Ways of Coping Inventory (Lazarus & Folkman, 1984) adapted for cancer patients, found that coping by seeking and using social support, focusing on the positive, and distancing was associated with less emotional distress. Interestingly, the specific cancer-related problem was not associated with how individuals coped but rather with their perception of the stress caused by the problem. Lichtman, Taylor, and Wood (1987) also found that supportive close relationships were related to adjustment, but one-fourth of the patients in their study reported at least one relationship in which communication was strained.

In a study of head and neck patients, Baker (1992) found that perceived social support was positively associated with a variety of measures of rehabilitation outcomes, including the psychosocial aspect. Zemore and Shepel (1989) found that breast cancer patients were no more emotionally distressed than were women with benign breast lumps or women in community samples, yet they reported

TABLE 1. Selected Studies on Social Support and Cancer (1987-93): Patient Populations, Measures Used, and Key Findings.

Baker, 1992. *Sample:* 52 patients with Stage II head and neck cancer. *Measure:* Personal Resources Questionnaire Part 2. *Findings:* Initial emotional upheaval associated with facial disfigurement did not impede the patients' rehabilitation. The psychosocial dimension (social interaction, communication, emotional behavior, and alertness) correlated with perceived social support.

Baron et al., 1990. *Sample:* 23 spouses of patients with mixed-stage renal, bladder, prostate, or testicular cancer. *Measure:* Social Provisions Scale. *Findings:* Spouses who had greater social support had faster T-cell proliferation when stimulated by the mitogen PHA, and their target tumor cells also were destroyed more effectively.

Dakof & Taylor, 1990. *Sample:* 55 patients with various late-stage cancers. *Measure:* Open-ended interview questions developed by the researchers. *Findings:* The victimization model applied more to interacting with nonfamily than family members. Support was found to be partially dependent on source: intimate others were most valued for emotional support, whereas physicians were valued primarily for informational support.

Dunkel-Schetter et al., 1992. *Sample:* 603 patients with mixed types and stages of cancer. *Measure:* Ways of Coping - CA. *Findings:* Site of cancer, time since diagnosis, or a specific cancer-related threat or problem were not associated significantly with coping. Coping through seeking and using social support, focusing on the positive, and distancing were associated with less emotional distress, whereas using cognitive and behavioral escape-avoidance was associated with more emotional distress.

Ell et al., 1989. *Sample:* 369 patients with early stage breast, colorectal, or lung cancer. *Measure:* Interview Schedule for Social Interaction, modified. *Findings:* Site and stage of illness were not associated with adequacy of support, but social integration was lowest among lung cancer patients. Social support was a significant predictor of psychological and functional adaptation, depending on the specific dimension of support, status of the patient's illness, and specific outcome.

Ell et al., 1992. *Sample:* 294 patients with mixed-stage breast, lung, or colorectal cancer. *Measure:* Interview Schedule for Social Interaction, modified. *Findings:* 220 patients survived. Emotional support provided by members of the primary social network was protective for survival during early stages of illness and for breast cancer.

Fawzy et al., 1993. *Sample:* 34 patients and 34 controls with Stage I or II melanoma. *Measure:* Dealing With Illness Coping Inventory. *Findings:* At 6 years, the control group had a significantly greater rate of death.

Feather & Wainstock, 1989a, 1989b. *Sample:* 933 breast cancer patients who completed questionnaires postsurgery; 27 participated in an open-ended interview. *Measure:* Norbeck Social Support Questionnaire. *Findings:* (1) Unmarried women living with a mate had lowest levels of support. Larger networks did not provide greater amounts of social support. Less well-educated women perceived greater emotional support than did better-educated women. Having friends was not related to emotional support. (2) Attitudes toward mastectomy were more strongly related to self-esteem than to social support, age, education, marital status, or adjuvant chemotherapy.

Gellert et al., 1993. *Sample:* 34 patients with mixed-stage breast cancer; 102 comparison patients. *Intervention:* Participation in Exceptional Cancer Patients program. *Findings:* Program participants did not live significantly longer than the control group.

Goodwin et al., 1991. *Sample:* 799 patients age 65 or older with newly diagnosed colon, rectal, breast, uterine, cervical, prostate, thyroid, or buccal cavity cancer or malignant melanoma. *Measure:* Questionnaire developed by the researchers. *Findings:* Need for support was often coupled with less than optimal social support networks. Risk factors for having poor social support networks included advanced age, non-Hispanic ethnicity, female sex, low income, and recent migration to the area (New Mexico residents).

Hilton, 1989. *Sample:* 227 patients with mixed-stage breast cancer. *Measure:* Revised Ways of Coping Scale. *Findings:* Women who perceived high uncertainty and uncontrollable life events and had a low commitment to life tended to use escape-avoidance instead of positive reappraisal strategies. Women who saw uncertain events as controllable tended to use planful problem solving, escape-avoidance, positive reappraisal, self-controlling strategies, and social support.

Irwin & Kramer, 1988. *Sample:* 181 patients with mixed cancers in various stages. *Measure:* Sustained Social Support Index. *Findings:* Patients with more socioemotional support also seemed less psychologically distressed. Distress from depressive symptoms declined among patients in the posttreatment period, but sustained social support had little independent effect on this amelioration.

Levy et al., 1990a. *Sample:* 66 patients with Stage I or II breast cancer 3 months postsurgery. *Measures:* Social support measure developed by Northouse (1988); Ways of Coping Checklist–revised. *Findings:* Seeking social support and perception of the quality of support received from significant others, particularly from a spouse or intimate other, were predictors of natural killer-cell activity, suggesting a stress-buffering role for this factor. However, the largest amount of variance in this activity was explained by tumor estrogen receptor values.

TABLE 1 (continued)

Levy et al., 1990b. *Sample:* 60 patients with Stage I or II breast cancer within 2 weeks of hospital discharge. *Measures:* A social support measure developed by Northouse (1988); Ways of Coping Checklist–revised. *Findings:* Patients' perception of the quality of emotional support received from significant others was the most important predictor of natural killer-cell activity. The tumor's estrogen receptor status was less important.

Litchtman et al., 1987. *Sample:* 78 patients with mixed-stage breast cancer. *Measures:* Questions developed by the researchers; Locke-Wallace Marital Adjustment Test. *Findings:* Supportive close relationships were associated with positive adjustment. One-fourth had at least one troubled relationship. Successful marital adjustment was associated with the husband's satisfaction with the relationship before cancer, when the wife's surgery was less severe, and when the husband acted supportive after her cancer.

Manne et al., 1990. *Sample:* 23 patients aged 3-9 with mixed cancers in various stages; 10 nurses. *Measure:* Procedure Behavior Rating Scale. *Findings:* Behavioral intervention incorporating parental coaching, attentional distraction, and positive reinforcement markedly reduced the child's behavioral distress, the parents' anxiety, and their ratings of the child's pain. Intervention did not influence children's perceptions of their own pain or nurses' ratings of their pain and distress.

Mishel & Braden, 1988. *Sample:* 61 patients with mixed-stage cervical, uterine, endometrial, vaginal, vulvar, or ovarian cancer. *Measure:* Norbeck Social Support Questionnaire. *Findings:* Social support, in the form of affirmation or sharing thoughts and ideas with others, had both an indirect and a direct impact on reducing uncertainty.

Neuling & Winefield, 1988. *Sample:* 58 postsurgical breast cancer patients. *Measure:* Multidimensional Support Scale. *Findings:* Frequency of support declined with time from surgery. Patients required empathic support from all sources, whereas they required informational support from surgeons, not family and friends. During hospitalization, lower anxiety and depression were related to satisfaction with support from family members. One month after surgery, anxiety and depression were related to satisfaction with support from surgeons; 3 months after surgery, anxiety and depression were related to satisfaction with support from family members and surgeons.

Northouse, 1988. *Sample:* 50 patients with Stage I or II breast cancer and their husbands. *Measure:* Social Support Questionnaire. *Findings:* Psychological distress was related to social support for both patients and husbands.

Rose, 1990. *Sample:* 64 patients with mixed cancers in various stages. *Measure:* Desired Support Questionnaire. *Findings:* Emotional and instrumental functions of support were independent. Distinctiveness of primary network members was manifested by patients' overall preference for tangible aid from family members, modeling from friends who had cancer, and open communication with and clarification from health professionals.

Speechley & Noh, 1992. *Sample:* 63 Parents of cancer survivors (63 mothers, 49 fathers) and a matched sample of parents of healthy children (64 mothers, 62 fathers). *Measure:* Provision of Social Relations Scale. *Findings:* Parents of children who survived cancer and experienced a lower degree of social support were more depressed than the normative samples.

Spiegel et al., 1989. *Sample:* 50 patients with Stage I-IV breast cancer; 36 controls. *Intervention:* Participation in a weekly support group for 1 year. *Findings:* Group participants survived significantly longer than controls.

Taylor et al., 1986. *Sample:* 667 patients with mixed cancers in various stages. *Measure:* Survey questionnaire developed by the researchers. *Findings:* Inadequate or unavailable social support from family, friends, and medical caregivers may be only modestly related to joining a support group. Individuals who were more likely to turn to support groups also appeared to have turned to a variety of other sources.

Tempelaar et al., 1989. *Sample:* 201 nonpatients, 109 surgery patients, and 108 chemotherapy patients with mixed cancers in various stages. *Measure:* Questionnaire developed by the researchers. *Findings:* Recently diagnosed patients who had undergone surgery or chemotherapy had more positive social experiences and fewer negative ones than did the random sample of nonpatients. Stigmatization and victimization were no more evident in the patient groups than in the control group. Positive social experiences were associated with a greater feeling of self-esteem; negative experiences were associated with neuroticism.

Vinokur & Vinokur-Kaplan, 1990. *Sample:* 431 patients with mixed-stage breast cancer. *Measure:* Interview questions developed by the researchers. *Findings:* Long-term survivors gave more social support to their husbands than they received. Husbands of recently diagnosed patients reported giving more social support to their wives than they received (the wives corroborated this). Wives in both samples reported engaging in more social undermining of others than they received. No associations were found in either group between wives' degree of physical impairment and social support received.

Ward et al., 1991. *Samples:* (1) 81 patients with mixed-stage lymphoma or nonmetastatic or metastatic breast cancer. (2) 78 patients with mixed cancers in various stages. *Measures:* Questionnaires developed by the researchers (some items were based on the Norbeck Social Support Questionnaire). *Findings:* (1) Patients who communicated more about cancer had lower self-esteem. (2) In the replication study, higher levels of communication were associated with greater self-esteem when information about treatment, side effects, and self-esteem was given to patients and significant others.

TABLE 1 (continued)

Waxler-Morrison et al., 1991. *Sample:* 133 patients with Stage I-IV breast cancer who completed questionnaires; 18 who were interviewed. *Measures:* Two self-administered questionnaires developed by the researchers, including a measure of social network; open-ended interview questions. *Finding:* Patients' social context, especially friendship and work outside the home, were statistically important for survival.

Williams, 1992. *Sample:* 17 primary caretakers of 15 children with mixed cancers in various stages; 33 health care professionals. *Measure:* Social Network Inventory, modified; in-depth interviews. *Finding:* Both health care professionals and parents defined support as including compassion; health care professionals also included knowledge.

Zemore & Shepel, 1989. *Sample:* 301 patients with Stage I or II breast cancer; 100 women with benign breast lumps. *Measure:* Social Adjustment Scale. *Findings:* Patients were no more maladjusted than the controls or a normative sample. They reported greater emotional support from family and friends than did controls. Those who said they were able to talk about their feelings and problems with a friend, relative, or spouse scored higher on adjustment than did those who said they were unable to confide in others.

that adjustment was related to the ability to confide in supportive others.

Northouse (1988) reported that psychological distress was related to social support for both the patient and the significant other. Vinokur and Vinokur-Kaplan (1990) explored the complexities of the perceptions of breast cancer patients and their husbands involving the giving and receiving of support and found that long-term survivors reported that they gave more assistance to their husband than they received from him. However, in their sample of recently diagnosed patients, husbands reported giving more support to their wife than they received (their perceptions were corroborated by wives' reports). The most striking finding was the lack of association between the wives' degree of physical impairment and the amount of social support they gave and received. The authors suggested that the fact of having a life-threatening illness itself may be sufficient for the husband to provide support. However, most patients in their sample did not have advanced disease (70 percent

had no nodal involvement); thus, the impact of a worsening prognosis on support remains unclear.

Irwin and Kramer (1988) highlighted the importance of disease
status as a variable that has an impact on the relationship between
social support and adjustment. Although they found that patients
who had more socioemotional support seemed to be less distressed,
they noted that depression declined in the posttreatment period and
that sustained social support had little independent effect on this
decline.

Ell et al. (1989), in a study of breast, colorectal, and lung cancer
patients, used a modified version of the Interview Schedule for
Social Interaction and found that social support was a significant
predictor of psychological and functional adaptation. However,
they also found that personal control may be more important than
support as a resource for reducing psychological distress and that
social resources provide an additional coping aid.

Mishel and Braden (1988) found that social support was a major
factor in reducing the uncertainty (i.e., ambiguity, complexity, lack
of information, and unpredictability) associated with having an illness. In a study of breast cancer patients, Hilton (1989) found that
women who see uncertain events as controllable use social support
along with planful problem solving, escape-avoidance, positive
appraisal, and self-controlling strategies to cope with a breast cancer diagnosis. However, Hilton did not measure the impact on psychological distress.

Several researchers have pursued the relationship between social
support and self-esteem. Feather and Wainstock (1989b) used the
Norbeck Social Support Questionnaire (Norbeck, Lindsey, & Carrieri, 1983) and found that attitudes of breast cancer patients toward
mastectomy were related more strongly to self-esteem than to social
support. Interestingly, in an earlier study, Feather and Wainstock
(1989a) reported that larger networks did not provide greater
amounts of social support.

In a study involving 81 cancer patients, Ward et al. (1991)
examined the relationship between social support, self-esteem, and
communication and found that patients perceived a high level of
social support. However, patients who communicated more about
the cancer had lower self-esteem. This finding was replicated in a

second study. The authors then introduced an information intervention and found that higher levels of communication were associated with greater self-esteem in the group receiving information that was given to both the patient and a significant other. Ward and colleagues suggested that shared information allowed patients to communicate their concerns without a corresponding loss of self-esteem.

It should be noted that there is increasing emphasis on the necessity of studying the impact of cancer, not only on the individual patient, but also on the entire family, which is generally the most intimate source of social support. A review of this literature is outside the scope of this article, but reviews can be found in Fobair and Zabora (this volume), Lewis (1993), Northouse and Peters-Golden (1993), and Sales, Schulz, and Biegel (1992).

In reviewing these studies, the following conclusions seemed clear:

- No consensus exists about the instruments that are most appropriate to measure social support or assess outcomes.
- Social support generally appears to be associated with psychosocial adaptation; however, it is unclear *how* this process occurs, for what types of patients, or at what stage of disease.

Social Support and Survival

Several studies have been undertaken to explore the complicated relationship between social support and survival. Ell et al. (1992) recently reported differential survival rates based on type of cancer for a sample of 294 patients studied at two and six months (74 patients had died). For patients with breast cancer, marital status was the only significant risk factor and emotional support was the only significant protective factor predicting survival. Stage of illness and role limitations were the only predictors of survival for patients with lung and colorectal cancer. An examination of the relationship between support and stage of illness showed that role limitations and adequacy of emotional support significantly predicted survival among patients with localized disease. Only stage of illness predicted survival among patients with more advanced disease.

Finally, Waxler-Morrison and colleagues (1991) examined a

cohort of 133 women with breast cancer to explore the relationship between social contexts at diagnosis and survival. Several measures of support were predictive of survival after accounting for extent of disease. The generalizability of these findings is limited because only 1 percent of the patients had metastatic disease and only 19 percent had local advanced disease. Almost all patients in the study had a modified radical mastectomy (uncommon today), and the authors did not mention the treatment the various groups of patients had received.

Several studies have examined the impact of membership in a support group on survival (although none of the studies was designed to answer that specific question). Gellert, Maxwell, and Siegel (1993) investigated Siegel's Exceptional Cancer Patients Group and found no increase in survival among group participants versus nonparticipants.

Two studies reported longer survival among group participants compared with controls. Spiegel et al. (1989) found that breast cancer patients in their treatment group lived significantly longer than did controls; however, no data on medical treatment during the intervention were reported. Fawzy et al. (1993) reported a significantly better survival rate among melanoma patients who attended a six-session treatment group, suggesting that the intervention may have fostered greater knowledge of health habits or possibly may have facilitated effective coping through discussion of similar problems.

Although several studies of immune function as a surrogate for improved outcome have been conducted, any conclusions from those studies are premature. In a study of spouses of cancer patients, Baron et al. (1990) suggested that social support improved the immune function of spouses of cancer patients independently of its effect on depression or negative life events. The authors made no attempt to control for the extraordinarily different outcomes among patients whose spouses were studied. The intensity of stress in the spouse of a young patient receiving chemotherapy for testicular cancer (with a more than 90 percent chance of cure) is distinctly different from the stress associated with the end stages of disease. Furthermore, a sample size of only 23 is insufficient to draw any strong conclusions.

Levy et al. (1990a, 1990b) attempted to link natural killer-cell activity to survival of breast cancer patients and, in turn, to perceptions of positive social support. A series of correlative interpretations was required to complete this journey, and no data were given concerning actual survival as it related to support or immune function. Baron et al. (1990), citing Calabrese, Kling, and Gold (1987), noted the lack of clear evidence that any variation in immunologic function, whether or not it is caused by increased social support, has any practical significance in altering health outcomes.

Goodwin, Hunt, and Samet (1991) noted that little is known about the social support of elderly persons. Given the high prevalence of illness and other stressors in this population, they suggested that support may play an important role in determining the outcome of illness in the elderly. These authors studied functional status and availability of social support networks among 799 elderly men and women in six New Mexico counties who had recently been diagnosed with cancer. The predictors of having a poor social support network included non-Hispanic white ethnicity, advanced age, low income, and being a recent migrant. Patients with functional limitations were more likely than other patients to have weak support networks. The combination of impaired functional status and a limited social support network, they concluded, may help to explain why elderly patients are at increased risk for not receiving appropriate medical treatment.

Support from Health Care Professionals

Dakof and Taylor's (1990) study of cancer patients' perceptions of helpful and unhelpful actions from providers of support revealed that the type of support patients desired varied across provider categories. Physicians were valued most for the information they provided; the absence of such information was sorely missed by patients. In contrast, patients identified esteem and emotional support as the most helpful types of support provided by nurses.

In a longitudinal study of patients' recovery after surgery for breast cancer, Neuling and Winefield (1988) found that the frequency of support declined over time after surgery. Type of support was related to source of support in that patients required informational aid from surgeons, not from family and friends, whereas they desired empathic support from all sources. Those who were satisfied with support from family members were less anxious and depressed during their hospitalization. At one month postsurgery, lower levels of anxiety and depression were related to satisfaction with support from surgeons, whereas lower levels of anxiety and depression were related to satisfaction with support from family members and surgeons three months postsurgery.

Rose (1990) also found that patients' preferences for some specific components of emotional support (i.e., desire for reassurance and esteem) were similar across the sources of support, which included family, friends, and health care professionals. Patients differed in their desire for the component of "open communication," with patients expressing a greater desire for "open communication" with their health care professionals, as compared with family or friends. When Rose examined the components of instrumental support, she found that patients consistently desired "directive guidance" and "advocacy" across sources. However, receiving "clarification" from the health care professional was more desirable than receiving it from other sources of support. Rose commented that although the patients' desire for "clarification" was expected, given the health care professional's expert role, their desire for "open communication" was surprising. She argued that the prominence patients gave to "open communication" may have been the result of difficulties they already may have experienced in communicating with their health care professionals. A second interesting finding involved the impact of the patients' perception of their prognosis. Those who perceived a poorer prognosis expressed a stronger desire for both instrumental and emotional support than did patients who perceived a more positive prognosis.

Taylor et al.'s survey (1986) of patients who attended and did not attend cancer support groups found that both positive and negative experiences in patient communication with the medical community influenced participation in support groups. A majority of the small segment of respondents who asked their physician or other medical personnel about joining a support group said they had been encouraged to participate. Those who did attend a support group were significantly more likely than nonattenders to report a negative experience with the medical community during their cancer episode. The authors speculated that perhaps a negative experience motivated these particular patients to seek out support and thus join a group. Interestingly, those who have turned to groups also have turned to a variety of other sources of support.

Williams (1992) compared the definition and description of social support held by parents of children with cancer with those held by oncology health care providers. Parents defined support as compassion, skill in listening, and caring. Health care providers defined it in terms of availability, levels of knowledge, and communication. Health care professionals identified the following as important supportive actions: being available, being consistent with the family, showing oneself as supportive, understanding and supporting the parental role, and assisting with needed resources. Williams argued that perceptions of support should be regarded as an important component of family assessment and that additional research is needed concerning factors that may alter parents' perceptions of support.

Feather and Wainstock's work (1989a, 1989b) with breast cancer patients after surgery found that 82 percent did not identify a health care professional as part of their support network. Patients who reported receiving support from their health care professionals, counselors, or both had a lower level of overall emotional support than did those who reported that their support network did not include health care providers. The authors suggested that "this could reflect physical and/or emotional problem needs among those seeking additional assistance" (p. 295).

Two issues are clear from this segment of the literature. First, closer consideration of the role of support in the relationship between health care professional and patient is warranted. Second, studies should be more specific about the categories of health care professionals who are considered to be sources of social support. The research of Neuling and Winefield (1988), Dakof and Taylor (1990), and Rose (1990) clearly indicated that the source of support considered interacts with type of support desired, whereas the work of Taylor et al. (1986) drew attention to the impact that such support, or the lack of support, may have on patients' participation in support groups. Williams's research (1992) highlighted potentially important differences in perceptions between those receiving and those giving social support, whereas Feather and Wainstock's studies (1989a, 1989b) showed the importance of individual differences in patients' needs. With the exception of the studies by Neuling and Winefield (1988) and Dakof and Taylor (1990), the specific type of professionals considered in this body of research is only globally defined, which leaves unaddressed the finer nuances that may be attributable to sources of support. Future research concerning social support in the relationship between the health care professional and the patient would be enhanced if issues concerning sources of support were identified and investigated more carefully.

Childhood Cancer

Finally, support has been found to be an important resource for parents of children with cancer. Speechley and Noh (1992) reported that parents of children who survived cancer and received low levels of social support were more depressed and anxious than was a matched sample of parents of healthy children. Manne et al. (1990) found that communication behaviors that included parental coaching, attentional distraction, and positive reinforcement were supportive strategies associated with decreased behavioral distress in children who were undergoing painful treatment procedures.

CONCLUSIONS AND FUTURE DIRECTIONS

The literature demonstrates support for the theoretical approach suggested by Thoits (1986) and expanded by Dunkel-Schetter et al. (1992) that social support is a coping strategy that patients use to reduce the stress accompanying the diagnosis of cancer and its treatment. Studies have generally been cross-sectional and have used a diverse set of assessment tools to measure social networks (e.g., numbers, sources) or the function of support or assistance provided, particularly informational or expressive aid.

Researchers do not agree on the contribution of social support to the reduction of stress and indeed use a variety of outcome instruments to measure psychosocial adaptation. The work of Matt and Dean (1993) described earlier raises the important question of the direction of the support-to-distress relationship and provides evidence that depressed mood and support may interact. Clearly, this question requires additional investigation. Studies are underway to test further and possibly explain the relationship between participation in a support group and survival reported by Spiegel et al. (1989) and Fawzy et al. (1993).

We now return to Albrecht and colleagues' suggestion that studies are needed that focus on the nature of the communication process in which support occurs–that is, on *how* social support is given and received (Albrecht & Adelman, 1987; Albrecht, Burleson, & Goldsmith, 1994). These studies would include an analysis of the messages exchanged, the mutually interdependent behaviors that occur, the nature of relationships (formal/informal, close/distant, and roles), the risks and benefits to the participants, the past history of relations between the parties, and, importantly, the type of support needed and perceived. Longitudinal studies are needed to examine the impact of disease stage on the interaction. The extent of agreement between patients and significant others regarding an evaluation of the supportive transaction needs to be explored. We predict that congruence between the providers' and recipients' perceptions of a successful exchange would be related to recipients' psychosocial adaptation. The selection of outcome measures of psychosocial adaptation should continue to be explored, drawing on quality-of-life instruments, because it seems logical that supportive transactions would influence many aspects of life in addition to mood.

In addition, how seeking and using social supports relates to the use of other coping strategies remains to be studied. Another arena for study is the impact of changes in the patient's social network. For example, work in progress by Blanchard and colleagues has found that a brief intervention aimed at reducing the distress of patients' spouses is associated with a decrease in patients' depression.

Finally, we expect that attempts to explain the process of support empirically will yield an understanding of how support enables patients and their significant others to cope by increasing their sense of personal control and mastery. This will enable them to manage better the profound uncertainty that accompanies the cancer experience.

REFERENCES

Albrecht, T. L., & Adelman, M. B. (1987). *Communicating social support.* Newbury Park, CA: Sage Publications.

Albrecht, T. L., Burleson, B. R., & Goldsmith, D. (1994). Supportive communication. In M. L. Knapp, & G. R. Miller (Eds.), *Handbook of interpersonal communication* (rev. ed., pp. 419-449). Newbury Park, CA: Sage Publications.

Baker, C. A. (1992). Factors associated with rehabilitation in head and neck cancer. *Cancer Nursing, 15,* 395-400.

Baron, R. S., Cutrona, C. E., Hicklin, D., Russell, D. W., & Lubaroff, D. M. (1990). Social support and immune function among spouses of cancer patients. *Journal of Personality & Social Psychology, 59,* 344-352.

Broadhead, W. E., & Kaplan, B. H. (1991). Social support and the cancer patient: Implications for future research and clinical care. *Cancer, 67*(Suppl. 3), 794-799.

Burleson, B. R., Albrecht, T. L., & Sarason, I. G. (Eds.) (1994). *Communication of social support.* Newbury Park, CA: Sage Publications.

Calabrese, J. R., Kling, M. A., & Gold, P. W. (1987). Alterations in immunocompetence during stress, bereavement, and depression: Focus on neuroendocrine regulation. *American Journal of Psychiatry, 144,* 1123-1134.

Cohen, S., & Syme, S. L. (Eds.) (1985). *Social support and health.* New York: Academic Press.

Cohen, S., & Wills, T. A. (1985). Stress, social support, and the buffering hypothesis. *Psychological Bulletin, 98,* 310-357.

Dakof, G. A., & Taylor, S. E. (1990). Victims' perceptions of social support: What is helpful from whom? *Journal of Personality & Social Psychology, 58*(1), 80-89.

Dunkel-Schetter, C., Feinstein, L. G., Taylor, S. E., & Falke, R. L. (1992). Patterns of coping with cancer. *Health Psychology, 11*(2), 79-87.

Ell, K. O., Mantell, J. E., Hamovitch, M. B., & Nishimoto, R. H. (1989). Social support, sense of control, and coping among patients with breast, lung, or colorectal cancer. *Journal of Psychosocial Oncology, 7*(3), 63-87.

Ell, K., Nishimoto, R., Mediansky, L., Mantell, J., & Hamovitch, M. (1992). Social relations, social support and survival among patients with cancer. *Journal of Psychosomatic Research, 36,* 531-541.

Fawzy, F. I., Fawzy, N. W., Hyun, C. S., Elashoff, R., Guthrie, D., Fahey, J. L., & Morton, D. L. (1993). Malignant melanoma: Effects of early structured psychiatric intervention, coping, and affective state on recurrence and survival 6 years later. *Archives of General Psychiatry, 50,* 681-689.

Feather, B. L., & Wainstock, J. M. (1989a). Perceptions of postmastectomy patients. Part I: The relationships between social support and network providers. *Cancer Nursing, 12,* 293-300.

Feather, B. L., & Wainstock, J. M. (1989b). Perceptions of postmastectomy patients. Part II: Social support and attitudes towards mastectomy. *Cancer Nursing, 12,* 301-309.

Gellert, G. A., Maxwell, R. M., & Siegel, B. S. (1993). Survival of breast cancer patients receiving adjunctive psychosocial support therapy: A 10-year follow-up study. *Journal of Clinical Oncology, 11*(1), 66-69.

Goodwin, J. S., Hunt, W. C., & Samet, J. M. (1991). A population-based study of functional status and social support networks of elderly patients newly diagnosed with cancer. *Archives of Internal Medicine, 151*, 366-370.

Hilton, A. (1989). The relationship of uncertainty, control, commitment, and threat of recurrence to coping strategies used by women diagnosed with breast cancer. *Journal of Behavioral Medicine, 12*(1), 39-54.

Irwin, P. H., & Kramer, S. (1988). Social support and cancer: Sustained emotional support and successful adaptation. *Journal of Psychosocial Oncology, 6*(1/2), 53-73.

Lazarus, R. S., & Folkman, S. (1984). *Stress, appraisal, and coping.* New York: Springer Publishing.

Levy, S. M., Herberman, R. B., Lee, J., Whiteside, T., Kirkwood, J., & McFeeley, S. (1990a). Estrogen receptor concentration and social factors as predictors of natural killer cell activity in early-stage breast cancer patients. *Natural Immunity & Cell Growth Regulation, 9*, 313-324.

Levy, S. M., Herberman, R. B., Whiteside, T., Sanzo, K., Lee, J., & Kirkwood, J. (1990b). Perceived social support and tumor estrogen/progesterone receptor status as predictors of natural killer cell activity in breast cancer patients. *Psychosomatic Medicine, 52*(1), 73-85.

Lewis, F. M. (1993). Psychosocial transitions and the family's work in adjusting to cancer. *Seminars in Oncology Nursing, 9*, 127-129.

Lichtman, R. R., Taylor, S. E., & Wood, J. V. (1987). Social support and marital adjustment after breast cancer. *Journal of Psychosocial Oncology, 5*(3), 47-74.

Manne, S. L., Redd, W. H., Jacobsen, P. B., Gorfinkle, K., Schorr, O., & Rapkin, B. (1990). Behavioral intervention to reduce child and parent distress during venipuncture. *Journal of Consulting & Clinical Psychology, 58*, 565-572.

Matt, G. E., & Dean, A. (1993). Social support from friends and psychological distress among elderly persons: Moderator effects of age. *Journal of Health & Social Behavior, 34*, 187-200.

Mishel, M. H., & Braden, C. J. (1988). Finding meaning: Antecedents of uncertainty in illness. *Nursing Research, 37*(2), 98-103, 127.

Nelles, W. B., McCaffrey, R. J., Blanchard, C. G., & Ruckdeschel, J. C. (1991). Social supports and breast cancer: A review. *Journal of Psychosocial Oncology, 9*(2), 21-34.

Neuling, S. J., & Winefield, H. R. (1988). Social support and recovery after surgery for breast cancer: Frequency and correlates of supportive behaviors by family, friends, and surgeon. *Social Science & Medicine, 27*, 385-392.

Norbeck, J. S., Lindsey, A. M., & Carrieri, V. L. (1983). Further development of the Norbeck Social Support Questionnaire: Normative data and validity testing. *Nursing Research, 32*, 4-9.

Northouse, L. L. (1988). Social support in patients' and husbands' adjustment to breast cancer. *Nursing Research, 37*(2), 91-95.

Northouse, L. L., & Peters-Golden, H. (1993). Cancer and the family: Strategies to assist spouses. *Seminars in Oncology Nursing, 9,* 74-82.

Rose, J. H. (1990). Social support and cancer: Adult patients' desire for support from family, friends, and health professionals. *American Journal of Community Psychology, 18,* 439-464.

Sales, E., Schulz, R., & Biegel, D. (1992). Predictors of strain in families of cancer patients: A review of the literature. *Journal of Psychosocial Oncology, 10*(2), 1-26.

Speechley, K. N., & Noh, S. (1992). Surviving childhood cancer, social support, and parents' psychological adjustment. *Journal of Pediatric Psychology, 17*(1), 15-31.

Spiegel, D., Kraemer, H. C., Bloom, J. R., & Gottheil, E. (1989, October 14). Effect of psychosocial treatment on survival of patients with metastatic breast cancer. *Lancet,* 888-891.

Taylor, S. E., Falke, R. L., Shoptaw, S. J., & Lichtman, R. R. (1986). Social support, support groups, and the cancer patient. *Journal of Consulting & Clinical Psychology, 54,* 608-615.

Tempelaar, R., de Haes, J. C. J. M., de Ruiter, J. H., Bakker, D., van den Heuvel, W. J. A., & van Nieuwenhuijzen, M. G. (1989). The social experiences of cancer patients under treatment: A comparative study. *Social Science & Medicine, 29,* 635-642.

Thoits, P. (1986). Social support as coping assistance. *Journal of Consulting & Clinical Psychology, 54,* 416-423.

Vinokur, A. D., & Vinokur-Kaplan, D. (1990). "In sickness and in health": Patterns of social support and undermining in older married couples. *Journal of Aging & Health, 2,* 215-241.

Ward, S., Leventhal, H., Easterling, D., Luchterhand, C., & Love, R. (1991). Social support, self-esteem, and communication in patients receiving chemotherapy. *Journal of Psychosocial Oncology, 9*(1), 95-116.

Waxler-Morrison, N., Hislop, T. G., Mears, B., & Kan, L. (1991). Effects of social relationships on survival for women with breast cancer: A prospective study. *Social Science & Medicine, 33,* 177-183.

Williams, H. A. (1992). Comparing the perception of support by parents of children with cancer and by health professionals. *Journal of Pediatric Oncology Nursing, 9,* 180-186.

Wortman, C. B. (1984). Social support and the cancer patient: Conceptual and methodological issues. *Cancer, 53,* 2339-2360.

Wortman, C. B., & Dunkel-Schetter, C. (1979). Interpersonal relations and cancer. *Journal of Social Issues, 35,* 120-155.

Wortman, C. B., & Dunkel-Schetter, C. (1987). Conceptual and methodological issues in the study of social support. In A. Baum & J. Singer (Eds)., *Handbook of psychology and health* (pp. 63-108). Hillsdale, NJ: Lawrence Erlbaum.

Zemore, R., & Shepel, L. F. (1989). Effects of breast cancer and mastectomy on emotional support and adjustment. *Social Science & Medicine, 28,* 19-27.

Family Functioning
as a Resource Variable
in Psychosocial Cancer Research:
Issues and Measures

Patricia A. Fobair, MSW, MPH
James R. Zabora, MSW

SUMMARY. This article defines family functioning, reviews the development of measures of family functioning (FACES, FES, F-COPES, and Family APGAR), analyzes studies that have used selected measurements, discusses unresolved issues, and concludes with comments on family functioning as a resource variable in psychosocial research. The four measures of family functioning are useful in clinical research that examines how families facilitate patients' responses to the cancer experience. *[Article copies are available from The Haworth Document Delivery Service: 1-800-342-9678.]*

A diagnosis of cancer disrupts all aspects of a patient's life. Numerous variables influence each person's ability to adapt to the

Ms. Fobair is a Clinical Social Worker, Department of Clinical Social Work & Discharge Planning, Stanford University Hospital, 300 Pasteur Drive, H012, Stanford, CA 94305. Mr. Zabora is Director, Department of Patient and Family Services, The Johns Hopkins Oncology Center, Baltimore, MD.

[Haworth co-indexing entry note]: "Family Functioning as a Resource Variable in Psychosocial Cancer Research: Issues and Measures." Fobair, Patricia A., and James R. Zabora. Co-published simultaneously in the *Journal of Psychosocial Oncology* (The Haworth Medical Press, an imprint of The Haworth Press, Inc.) Vol. 13, No. 1/2, 1995, pp. 97-114; and: *Psychosocial Resource Variables in Cancer Studies: Conceptual and Measurement Issues* (ed: Barbara Curbow, and Mark R. Somerfield), The Haworth Medical Press, an imprint of The Haworth Press, Inc., 1995, pp. 97-114. *[Single or multiple copies of this article are available from The Haworth Document Delivery Service: 1-800-342-9678, 9:00 a.m.-5:00 p.m. (EST)]*.

illness and effectively resolve the many problems associated with the disease and its treatments. The importance of examining family functioning after a cancer diagnosis is becoming more apparent to clinicians who are concerned about their patients' quality of life after treatment (Lewis, Ellison, & Woods, 1985; Spiegel, Bloom, & Gottheil, 1983; Woods, Haberman, & Packard, 1993). Despite its importance, the family is often treated as a bystander rather than as an influential, organizing, and creative agent (Lewis, Ellison, & Woods, 1985). Family functioning can be an important resource for the patient–possibly more important than other forms of social support (Fobair et al., 1993; Lewis, Hammond, & Woods, 1993). Even though there are more than eight million cancer survivors in the United States (*Cancer Facts and Figures*, 1994), examination of family functioning is still a recent event in cancer research.

ROLE OF FAMILY FUNCTIONING IN RESEARCH

Early psychosocial cancer research focused on concerns related to the patient's well-being after treatment. More recently, researchers have sketched the psychological problems and role conflicts of family members (Germino & Funk, 1993; Lewis, Ellison, & Woods, 1985; Northouse, 1984; Wellisch et al., 1991a, 1991b). Although cancer has been viewed as a problem that involves the entire family, only recently have researchers examined variables and psychological outcomes systematically from the perspective of the patient's spouse and children or how family functioning serves as a resource for people with cancer. In this article, we will focus on the issues and measurements that relate to family functioning as a resource for people with cancer. Family functioning will be defined, the development of four measures of family functioning will be reviewed, and studies that have used selected measures will be discussed. Finally, unresolved issues and comments on the usefulness of family functioning as a resource for people with cancer will be presented.

DEFINITIONS AND MEASURES
OF FAMILY FUNCTIONING

Recent studies of how families respond to the stress of cancer cite the importance of family systems theory. As a result, the state of one family member influences the state of other members (Issel, Ersek, & Lewis, 1990), and the illness of one member reverberates through the entire family system (Northouse, 1984).

Family cohesion, flexibility, and communication are three terms used to describe marital and family dynamics (Olson, 1993). Family functioning can be viewed as the manner in which family members fulfill necessary roles and perform practical tasks that help the family live together and move ahead through time. Moos (1984) defined family functioning as how well family members relate to each other, pursue goals, organize activities, and accept family routines and procedures. Family functioning also can be viewed as the adjustments and adaptations that families experience as they move through the family life cycle (McCubbin et al., 1989).

Beginning with the central concepts of cohesion and adaptability defined by the early work of Angell (1936), the concept of family functioning has been expanded and refined with measurement scales that can detect various differences among families. The following are four important measures used in health research and in studies of patients with cancer. All of these measures incorporate aspects of family cohesion and adaptability in their design:

- Family Adaptability and Cohesion Evaluation Scale (FACES) (Olson, 1993).
- Family Environment Scale (FES) (Moos, 1974).
- Family Crisis Oriented Personal Evaluation Scale (F-COPES) (McCubbin et al., 1989).
- Family Adaptability, Partnership, Growth, Affection, Resolve Scale (Family APGAR) (Smilkstein, 1978).

Family Adaptability and Cohesion Evaluation Scale

Development. Olson, Sprenkle, and Russell (1979) developed FACES to measure two critical family constructs–adaptability and cohesion. Family adaptability, cohesion and communication were defined as the three dimensions of the Circumplex Model of marital and family systems. They defined *family cohesion* as the level of emotional bonding between family members and the degree of individual autonomy a person experiences in the family system. High family cohesion can be described as enmeshment, and low cohesion can be described as disengagement. Specific variables include emotional bonding, coalitions between parent and child, time, space, friends, decision-making, recreation, and other interests. *Family adaptability* is the ability of a marital or family system to change its power structure, role relationships, and relationship rules in response to situational and developmental stress. Highly adaptive families have the flexibility required to deal with changes in family roles and rules, whereas highly rigid families are hampered in their ability to change in response to such stress. Olson (1994) now describes behavior related to changes in family roles and rules as *flexibility* rather than adaptability.

Adaptability and cohesion can be used to identify 16 types of marital and family systems. When categorizing families, Olson and colleagues determined that well-functioning families had moderate scores on family adaptability and cohesion, whereas poorly functioning families had extreme scores on these two dimensions (Olson & Tiesel, 1993).

Although there are three versions of this instrument, FACES II is most often cited in psychosocial research. This 30-item self-report instrument is designed to determine family cohesion (16 items) and adaptability (14 items). Family members are asked to describe the behavior of other family members on a five-point Likert-type scale ("almost never" to "almost always"). Two items address each of the following dimensions of cohesion: emotional bonding, family boundaries, coalitions, time, space, friends, decision-making, interests and recreation. Two to three items measure each of the following dimensions of adaptability: assertiveness, leadership, discipline, negotiation, roles, and rules.

Scoring ranges for FACES II were developed on the basis of a national sample of families that included 2,453 adults and 412 adolescents. This normative sample represented all geographic regions throughout the United States. Although FACES III (the latest version) has been used in more than 500 research projects with good evidence of reliability and validity, recent findings suggest that FACES II has some advantages over FACES III. Although the test-retest reliabilities for FACES III are relatively high over a four-or five-week period (cohesion, .83; adaptability, .80), the Cronbach alphas are higher for FACES II (cohesion, .87 versus .77;

adaptability .78 versus .62). The higher alphas are a direct result of more items on the FACES II (30 versus 20 for FACES III). Furthermore, other instruments that measure constructs similar to cohesion and adaptability correlate higher with FACES II. As a result, Olson, Bell, and Portner (1992) recommended the use of FACES II for research and of FACES III for clinical work with patients.

Strengths. The high internal consistency of FACES II makes it a highly reliable measure that can be used both as a strong independent and as a dependent measure. With its clinical rating scale, the results can be used to validate the internal measure of functioning by external observations of family behavior. Approximately 30 studies involving cancer patients and their families using versions of FACES are in process (Olson, 1992).

Weaknesses. Horowitz and Kazak (1990) found that FACES II was unable to differentiate families that had a child with cancer from those that did not. Negative correlations between the results of the FACES and sibling adjustment raised concerns about the usefulness of the Circumplex Model in research on chronic childhood illnesses. Walker, McLaughlin, and Greene (1988) were unable to replicate the curvilinear relationships between family functioning and dimensions of the FACES. Recent reports also indicate difficulty in using FACES with traditional subgroups such as Hispanic families, for whom the concept of family adaptability is less relevant (e.g., Baker et al., 1995).

Concerns. Does the Circumplex Model create a value bias in the interpretation of high or extreme scores? Olson, Portner, and Bell (1982) believed that some extreme family types function in a positive manner. This hypothesis was particularly relevant for cultural groups with norms that support the extremes of family behavior (e.g., the rigidly enmeshed patterns observed in Mormon, Orthodox Jewish, and Amish families). Because empirical data suggest that FACES II does not capture the extremely high-scoring categories, Olson, Bell, and Portner (1992) cautioned readers to avoid using the terms enmeshed and chaotic and to reinterpret high scores on adaptability and cohesion as meaning "very connected" and "very flexible."

In sum, although the FACES II measures the essential family characteristics of cohesion and adaptability with high reliability, it has occasionally failed to differentiate between functional and non-functional families. This may suggest that a value bias exists concerning what constitutes a functional family (Olson, Bell, & Portner, 1992).

Family Environment Scale

Development. The FES was among the earliest self-report family assessment scales developed. Moos, Insel, and Humphrey (1974) formulated measures that assess the underlying characteristics of families, the work place, and social-and task-oriented groups. Moos and his colleagues believed that human behavior and adaptation could best be understood using a social ecology perspective: that is, social and physical environments have profound effects on human beings. Moos viewed a serious physical illness or injury as a life crisis and believed that a person's cognitive appraisal of the significance of the crisis might set forth basic adaptive tasks to which various coping skills could be applied. Because the crisis of cancer affects the patient's entire social environment, families must also respond to the challenges and stressors through adaptive tasks and coping skills. Family environment is one element in the social environment that contributes to the outcome of a crisis for the patient.

The FES consists of 10 subscales that measure the social-environmental characteristics of all types of families in three underlying domains: the *relationship domain,* measured by the Cohesiveness, Expressiveness, and Conflict subscales; the personal growth or goal orientation domain, measured by the Independence, Achievement Orientation, Intellectual-Cultural Orientation, Active-Recreational Orientation, and More Religious Emphasis subscales; and the *system maintenance domain*, measured by the Organization and Control subscales. The FES is available as either a 90-item or a 40-item true-false questionnaire. Normative data on the FES subscales were developed as a result of an analysis of 1,125 normal and 500 distressed families. This national sample of families was selected from all geographic regions of the country. Distressed families were selected from a variety of settings including psychiatric units, probation and parole departments and substance abuse clinics.

Finally, a frequently used 27-item composite scale, the Family Relationship Index (FRI), consists of three FES subscales: Cohesion, Expressiveness, and Conflict (Fobair et al., 1993; Spiegel, Bloom, & Gottheil, 1983; Vess, Moreland, & Schwebel, 1985). The Cronbach's alpha for this index is quite high at .89, which allows the FRI to be considered for use to measure the quality of support found in family relationships.

Strengths. The main strength of the FES is its usefulness as a snapshot of family functioning with many diverse groups of patients (Moos, 1984). The breadth and diversity of its content allows clinical researchers to tap into issues of independence and autonomy as well as four other areas of personal growth: achievement, intellectual-cultural, active-recreational, and moral-religious. With regard to the known groups validity (Robinson, Shaver, & Wrightsman, 1991) of the FES, more than 200 studies have demonstrated that the measure differentiates between different types of families and between distressed and nondistressed families (Moos, 1992). In addition, the true-false dichotomous response format makes the FES useful with patients who have mild cognitive impairments (Moos, 1990).

Although the measure is used to describe and compare family social environments, it probably is best known as a research tool in medical and educational settings. Among the more than 250 studies listed in the FES annotated bibliography (Moos, 1992), at least a dozen involve cancer patients.

Weaknesses. The FES is better known for its role in group research as an independent variable than for clinical evaluations of individual families. Although reliability coefficients above .70 are generally viewed as satisfactory, higher levels of reliability (.80 or higher) are recommended when the measure is to be used as a dependent measure. Many of the subscales have reliabilities ranging from .61 to .78 (Roosa & Beals, 1990). Moos (1990) identified two features that tend to lower the reliability coefficients. First, in an effort to measure broad family constructs, diverse items were selected and highly intercorrelated items were dropped to reduce redundancy. Second, the true-false dichotomous response format contributes to greater problems with internal consistency. Fewer dimensions and a multipoint response format would increase the internal consistency.

Concerns. The FES has also experienced problems in studies among ethnic populations. Although the measure was normed to include ethnic family characteristics, two studies reported low internal consistency among adult African-American and Mexican-American families (Baranowski et al., 1986) and Puerto Rican and Vietnamese foster families (Munet-Vilaro & Egan, 1990).

In sum, the FES can be useful for discriminating between different types of families. Given its broad and diverse content, it has a positive record. However, the diversity of its content and the true-false dichotomous response format contribute to lower alpha coefficients (Moos, 1990).

Family Crisis Oriented Personal Evaluation Scale

Development. McCubbin's model of family adjustment and adaptation comes from the tradition of theory and research linking illness to stress in daily life, particularly family life. The work based on the theories of Adolf Meyer (Lief, 1948), Holmes and Rahe (1967), and Patterson and McCubbin (1983) provides explanations for the variability in individual susceptibility to illness and disease. Families attempt to manage the illness-related demands, and their responses seek to achieve a balance in family functioning (i.e., adjustment and adaptation). The model of adaptation depicts the family as a reactor to stress and a manager of resources within the family system and considers three levels of family functioning: the individual, the family unit, and the community (Patterson & McCubbin, 1983).

McCubbin, Larsen, and Olson (1982) conceptualized family coping efforts in response to a defined stressor and developed F-COPES to measure and evaluate the performance of family members. Family coping is defined as the coordinated problem-solving behavior of the entire family. In this model, the impact of stress is mediated by how families appraise the stressful situation and how they manage it (Nolan et al., 1992). Family coping is a process of achieving a balance in the family system that facilitates organization and unity and promotes individual growth and development (Stetz, Lewis, & Primomo, 1986). Family homeostasis is maintained when the coping strategy the family selects enables members to meet the demands of the stressful event and promotes overall adaptation (Nolan et al., 1992).

The F-COPES is a 30-item Likert scale that measures family coping behaviors with eight subscales: (1) problem solving, (2) reframing, (3) passivity, (4) religious support, (5) consulting the extended family, (6) seeking help, (7) receiving help from neighbors, and (8) seeking professional help. Respondents indicate on a five-point scale (1 = Strongly agree, 5 = Strongly disagree) the extent to which they agree that each coping strategy describes their response to a given problem. Total scores range from 30 to 150, with a high score representing an increase in the number of coping strategies used. Normative data were collected from two groups: 119 graduate and undergraduate students at the University of Minnesota and 2,582 working professionals in the human services field. The overall Cronbach's alpha reliability coefficient is .77; the reliability of the subscales ranges from .62 to .83; and the test-retest reliability for the final scale is .81 (McCubbin, Olson, & Larsen, 1991).

Strengths. The F-COPES provides a useful systematic assessment of family problem solving, communication, and coping that has been a popular clinical tool for use with families and at-risk adolescents. In research, it is used primarily as an independent variable. The internal consistencies exceed .80 for three out of five subscales and .70 for four out of five of the test-retest alphas. Because the F-COPES focuses on how family units solve problems, it may provide insight concerning the family's ability to serve as a resource for the patient.

Weaknesses. All items on the F-COPES are framed in the positive direction, which creates the potential for a response bias. A lack of agreement continues regarding whether the F-COPES actually measures family coping or individual problem-solving. In addition, the measure may not be stable over time as treatment effects occur. Furthermore, the actual coping behaviors may be too narrowly defined and, as a result, may not be culturally sensitive.

Concerns. Stetz, Lewis, and Primomo (1986) described two limitations of the F-COPES. First, because the self-report format elicits information about a family's sense of direction or coping style, it fails to identify strategies used for specific problems. Second, because each family member is asked individually to identify a recent problem or challenge and to describe what coping responses they used, other family members do not always identify the same problem. Consequently, an aggregation of individual members' scores is difficult to achieve. Finally, interpretation of the total score may be unclear since all strategies (e.g., "Watching TV" versus "Seeking assistance from a community agency") are given equal weight.

Family APGAR

Development. The Family APGAR (Smilkstein, 1978) is useful in clinical work as a brief screening instrument for rapid identification of problem families and in research as a global measure of family functioning that relates social support to physical health outcomes (Smilkstein, Ashworth, & Montana, 1982). The measure consists of five questions that elicit information regarding satisfaction with family life: adaptability, partnership, growth, affection, and resolve. A three-choice format (2 = Almost always, 1 = Some of the time, and 0 = Hardly ever) is generally used. The sum of the responses yields scores ranging from 0 to 10. A score of 8-10 suggests a highly functional family, a score of 4-7 indicates moderate dysfunction, and a score of 0-3 is equated with severe dysfunction (Grotevant & Carlson, 1989).

The Family APGAR exhibits good internal consistency, with an alpha of .80 and interitem correlations of .65 and .67. This level of reliability is acceptable for such a brief measure. Its split-half reliability is .93, and its two-week test-retest reliability is .83. An expanded five-choice response format yields a higher alpha (.86). Construct and criterion validity were established through correlations with the Pless-Salter White Family Function Index, with a validity correlation of .80 (Smilkstein, Ashworth, & Montana, 1982).

In a study of 50 bone marrow transplant patients and their families, 16 families (32 percent) scored 6 or lower on the Family APGAR at the time of admission (Zabora et al., 1993); scores below 7 suggest moderate-to-severe dysfunction. These families may be the same families that exhibit problematic behaviors that the medical team finds difficult to manage (Zabora et al., 1989). Because the APGAR tends to create a situation in which family satisfaction is viewed as a dichotomous variable (i.e., high versus low family functioning), its greater usefulness may be in the clinical arena, where it can be used in psychosocial screening programs to quickly identify potentially problematic families.

Strengths. Although the Family APGAR has not been used in many cancer studies, its popularity is increasing. Psychosocial screening as families enter the cancer experience is a worthwhile activity that may prospectively identify the extent to which a family may serve as a resource to the patient (Zabora & Smith, 1991; Zabora et al., 1992). Smilkstein (1978) believed that this tool could be useful in identifying and evaluating the family's present and past crises as well as the level of family function and family resources. In many cases, psychosocial studies would benefit from a brief global measure of family functioning.

Weaknesses. Although the brevity of the measure is a benefit, the likelihood that the measure may be incapable of differentiating the significant amount of variability that exists within family systems and subsystems is increased. Also, further investigation is necessary to examine which response format is most appropriate for clinical research.

Concerns. A word of caution is necessary concerning the interpretation of the scores. Some evidence suggests that highly cohesive or enmeshed families may obtain a score of 8 to 10. Enmeshment may be indicative of extreme family dysfunction, and the Family Apgar may label such a family as highly functional (Groterant & Carlson, 1989).

FAMILY FUNCTIONING AS A RESOURCE VARIABLE

In Spiegel, Bloom, and Gottheil's study (1983) of family environment and its relationship to adjustment to metastatic breast cancer, 54 women were assessed using the FES. Mood was measured with the Profile of Mood States (POMS) (McNair, Lorr, & Droppleman, 1971). Patient's total mood disturbance was the dependent variable in a stepwise multiple regression analysis with the FES scores. Control variables were group treatment, survival, beliefs about cancer, and moral-religious orientation; expressiveness and conflict were used as predictors. More expressiveness and less conflict in the family were associated with less mood disturbance in the patient group. According to Spiegel and his colleagues, these findings indicated that the family is a crucial factor in patients' adjustment and that "conspiracies of silence" in the family may be harmful. Table 1 details significant components of this study and other investigations of family functioning as a resource variable.

FACES II has been used to examine family behavior during a patient's prolonged hospitalization for bone marrow transplantation (Zabora & Smith, 1991; Zabora et al., 1989). Although the families of most cancer patients develop collaborative relationships with the medical team, a minority present management problems. Zabora and colleagues identified the following six family behaviors that caused problems for the medical team: (1) interfering directly with medical treatment, (2) making excessive demands on the staff's

---

TABLE 1. Review of Studies with Family Functioning as a Resource Variable

---

Birenbaum & Robinson, 1991. *Sample*: 34 parents from 19 families whose child received terminal care at home and 27 parents from 18 families whose child died in the hospital. *Time of measurement*: Parents were assessed before the child's death and again 1 year after the death. *Psychometrics*: FES (FRI). Alphas ranged from .50 to .79.

Lewis, Hammond, & Woods, 1993. *Sample:* 40 families with a mother recently diagnosed with breast cancer. *Time of measurement:* First interview of a series over 18 months. *Psychometrics*: F-COPES, FACES II. Alphas .83.

Lewis et al., 1989. *Sample*: 48 fathers of children ages 6-12 whose wives had breast cancer, fibrocystic breast disease, or diabetes. *Time of measurement:* Second interview during a 3-year study. *Psychometrics*: F-COPES, FACES II. Alphas .84.

Primomo, Yates, & Woods, 1990. *Sample*: 125 women: 58 with breast cancer, 36 with fibrocystic breast disease, and 31 with diabetes. *Time of measurement*: Cross-sectional survey. Median time since treatment: 5 years. *Psychometrics*: FACES II. Alpha = .91.

Spiegel, Bloom, & Gottheil, 1983. *Sample*: 58 women with metastatic breast cancer. *Time of measurement*: 4 interviews over 1 year after baseline. *Psychometrics*: FES. Alphas unknown.

---

time, (3) refusing to comply with guidelines on the medical unit or encouraging the patient to be noncompliant, (4) forming alliances with other families against the staff, (5) using the staff inappropriately, (6) being unavailable to make decisions or provide support to the patient (Zabora & Smith, 1992). Clearly, family difficulties influenced the patients' ability to respond to treatment challenges and to plan for post-discharge care.

The work of Lewis and her colleagues using the F-COPES also demonstrates important results regarding family coping styles. In a study that focused on the mothers and their partners in 40 families, Lewis, Hammond, and Woods (1993) found that the family's coping behavior figured prominently as a predictor of family functioning for the patient and the partner. Families did better when they managed their problems by increasing the frequency with which they discussed the reasons for what they did and by offering feedback to each other regarding daily activities. This finding was consistent with their earlier results (Lewis et al., 1989), which indicated that families with higher levels of marital adjustment used reflective discussion and fathers communicated more often with their children. The result was higher levels of psychosocial functioning for the patient.

DISCUSSION

The four measures of family functioning discussed here were selected for review because they are often used and are expected to be the most useful measures of family functioning in the future. When each measure is understood in the context in which it was developed, its specific usefulness in research becomes apparent. For example, the FES was designed to determine the strengths of patients' family situations that would predict capacities to deal with life inside or outside a psychiatric treatment setting (Moos, 1974). Olson, Sprenkle, and Russell (1979) developed the Circumplex Model to bridge the gaps between theorists, researchers, and practitioners. FACES II is based on a richly developed theory of family functioning intended to aid practitioners in family therapy and to stimulate research (Olson, 1993). In psychosocial research, FACES II is used most often as a dependent variable. McCubbin and Patterson (1981) published the F-COPES to identify problem-solving and behavioral strategies that families use in difficult situations. The Family APGAR (Smilkstein, 1978; Smilkstein, Ashworth, & Montana, 1982) was developed to provide a practical evaluation tool of family function for use in clinical practice. It is a brief tool for health professionals who wish to survey a patient population to identify vulnerable dysfunctional families, which in turn may influence the ability of these families to serve as a resource for the patient.

Is there a best measure? After a review of the major family measures, McCubbin and colleagues found that the FACES II was useful in evaluating family typology, the FES was useful as a measure in evaluating family resources, the F-COPES was useful as a family coping and problem-solving tool, and the Family APGAR was useful for identifying and evaluating family crises (McCubbin & McCubbin, 1993; McCubbin et al., 1989). Each measure has a useful role to play, depending on the study design and the methodological requirements. FACES is useful as a dependent measure, whereas the FES has breadth and depth as an independent variable. F-COPES examines family coping as a useful independent measure, and the Family APGAR is a useful brief independent variable and clinical tool.

Further assessment and intervention studies are necessary to examine and understand the impact of family functioning on how patients adapt to the many stressors associated with the diagnosis of cancer and its related treatments. Intervention studies should examine services offered to families that reduce their distress and improve their behavioral adjustment. In addition, studies are needed that determine the family's impact on the patient beyond the acute phases of cancer to include recurrence and terminal care. Finally, these studies must include ethnically, economically, and culturally diverse families (Lewis, Hammond, & Woods, 1993).

CONCLUSIONS

Examination of family functioning and its impact on the psychological adaptation of patients remains a recent event in cancer research. The family can act as a buffer against the problems of illness for the cancer patient. However, in a small percentage of families, changes in functioning over time may leave the patient feeling overly immersed in, or disengaged from, family relationships. Although family functioning can be an important resource for the patient, it can also be a source of distress.

The four measures of family functioning reviewed here can be used for both clinical and research purposes. Each one draws on a concept of family functioning that includes family cohesion, flexibility, and communication processes and how each of these dimensions helps or hinders the ongoing adjustment of cancer patients as they progress across the continuum of care from diagnosis to treatment and on to survivorship.

It is hoped that investigators will consider these issues before selecting a measure for clinical or research work with cancer patients. Three measures (FACES, FES, and F-COPES) originated in active and dynamic research centers where refinements of the measures are a part of the process. Indeed, it seems to be the nature of psychosocial measurement that new experiences in the field set directions for future research.

REFERENCES

Angell, R. (1936). *The family encounters the depression.* New York: Charles Scribner's Sons.

Baker, F., Zabora, J. R., Douglas, J. Y., & Jodrey, D. B. (1995, March 1). Measurement of qualities of life in special populations. Paper presented at the NCI Investigators' Meeting, Bethesda, MD.

Baranowski, T., Dworkin, R. J., Hooks, P., Nader, P. R., & Brown, J. (1986). The reliability of two measures of family functioning in three ethnic groups. *Family Perspective, 20,* 353-364.

Birenbaum, L., & Robinson, M. A. (1991). Family relationships in two types of terminal care. *Social Science & Medicine, 12,* 95-102.

Cancer facts and figures. (1994). Atlanta, GA: American Cancer Society.

Fobair, P., Bloom, J., Kuspa, L., Varghese, A., & Spiegel, D. (1993, April 22). The role of family support in patient adaptation to Hodgkin's disease. Paper presented at the annual meeting of the Association of Oncology Social Workers, New York, NY.

Germino, B. B., & Funk, S. G. (1993). Impact of a parent's cancer on adult children: Role and relationship issues. *Seminars in Oncology Nursing, 9*(2), 101-106.

Grotevant, H. D., & Carlson, C. I. (1989). *Family assessment: A guide to methods & measures.* New York: Guilford Press.

Hilton, B. A. (1993). Issues, problems, and challenges for families coping with breast cancer. *Seminars in Oncology Nursing, 9*(2), 88-100.

Holmes, T. H., & Rahe, R. (1967). The Social Readjustment Rating Scale. *Journal of Psychosomatic Research, 11*, 213-218.

Horowitz, W. A., & Kazak, A. E. (1990). Family adaptation to childhood cancer: Sibling and family systems variables. *Journal of Clinical Child Psychology, 19*, 221-228.

Issel, L. M., Ersek, M., & Lewis, F. M. (1990). How children cope with mother's breast cancer. *Oncology Nursing Forum, 17*(3), 5-13.

Lewis, F. M., Ellison, E. S., & Woods, N. F. (1985). The impact of breast cancer on the family. *Seminars in Oncology Nursing, 1*, 206-213.

Lewis, F. M., Hammond, M. A., & Woods, N. F. (1993). The family's functioning with newly diagnosed breast cancer in the mother: The development of an explanatory model. *Journal of Behavioral Medicine, 16*, 351-370.

Lewis, F. M., Woods, N. F., Hough, E. E., & Bensley, L. S. (1989). The family's functioning with chronic illness in the mother: The spouse's perspective. *Social Science & Medicine, 29*, 1261-1269.

Lief, A. (Ed.). (1948). *The common sense psychiatry of Dr. Adolf Meyer.* New York: McGraw-Hill.

McCubbin, M. A., & McCubbin, H. I. (1993). Families coping with illness: The resiliency model of family stress, adjustment and adaptation. In C. Danielson, B. Hamel-Bissell, & P. Winstead-Fry (Eds.), *Families, health and illness* (pp. 21-63). St. Louis: C. V. Mosby.

McCubbin, H. I., & Patterson, J. M. (1981). *Systematic assessment of family stress, resources and coping: Tools for research, education and clinical intervention.* St. Paul: University of Minnesota, Department of Family Social Science.

McCubbin, H. I., Larsen, A., & Olson, D. (1982). F-COPES: Family Crisis Oriented Personal Scales. In McCubbin & A. I. Thompson (Eds.), *Family assessment inventories for research and practice* (pp. 194-207). Madison: University of Wisconsin Press.

McCubbin, H. I., Olson, D. H., & Larsen, A. S. (1991). F-COPES: Family Crisis Oriented Personal Evaluation Scales. In McCubbin & A. I. Thompson (Eds.), *Family assessment inventories for research and practice* (2nd ed., pp. 203-214). Madison: University of Wisconsin Press.

McCubbin, H. I., McCubbin, M. A., Thompson, A. I., & Huang, S. T. T. (1989). Family assessment and self-report instruments in family medicine research. In C. N. Ramsey, Jr. (Ed.), *Family systems in medicine* (pp. 181-214). New York: Guilford Press.

McNair, D. M., Lorr, M., & Droppleman, L. F. (1971). *Profile of Mood States.* San Diego: Educational and Industrial Testing Service.

Moos, R. H. (1974). *Evaluating treatment environments: A social ecological approach.* New York: John Wiley & Sons.

Moos, R. H. (1984). *Coping with physical illness. 1. New perspectives.* New York: Plenum Medical Book.

Moos, R. H. (1990). Conceptual empirical approaches to developing family-based assessment procedures: Resolving the case of the Family Environment Scale. *Family Process, 29,* 199-208.

Moos, R. H. (1992). *Family Environment Scale: An annotated bibliography.* Palo Alto, CA: Consulting Psychologists Press.

Moos, R. H., Insel, P. M., & Humphrey, B. (1974). *Preliminary manual for the family, work, and group environment scales.* Palo Alto, CA: Consulting Psychologists Press.

Munet-Vilaro, F., & Egan, M. (1990). Reliability issues of the Family Environment Scale for cross-cultural research. *Nursing Research, 39,* 244-247.

Nolan, M. T., Cupples, S. A., Brown, M. M., Pierce, L., Lepley, D., & Ohler, L. (1992). Perceived stress and coping strategies among families of cardiac transplant candidates during the organ waiting period. *Heart & Lung, 21,* 540-547.

Northouse, L. (1984). The impact of cancer on the family: An overview. *International Journal of Psychiatric Medicine, 14,* 215-242.

Olson, D. H. (1991). *FACES II: Linear scoring & interpretation.* St. Paul: University of Minnesota, Department of Family Social Science.

Olson, D. H. (1992, January). *Published studies using FACES.* Unpublished document, University of Minnesota, Department of Family Social Science, St. Paul.

Olson, D. H. (1993). Circumplex Model of marital and family systems: Assessing family functioning. In F. Walsh-Froma (Ed.), *Normal family processes* (pp. 104-137). New York: Guilford Press.

Olson, D. H. (1994). Curvilinearity survives: The world is not flat. *Family Process, 33,* 471-478.

Olson, D. H., & Tiesel, J. W. (1993). *Assessment of family functioning: Diagnostic sourcebook* (Workshop on Family Data and Family Health Policy Proceedings). Washington, DC: National Institute on Drug Abuse.

Olson, D. H., Bell, R., & Portner, J. (1992). *FACES II.* St. Paul: University of Minnesota, Department of Family Social Science.

Olson, D. H., Portner, J., & Bell, R. Q. (1982). *FACES II: Family Adaptability and Cohesion Evaluation Scales.* St. Paul: University of Minnesota, Department of Family Social Science.

Olson, D. H., Sprenkle, C. H., & Russell, C. S. (1979). Circumplex Model of marital and family systems: I. Cohesion and adaptability dimensions, family types, and clinical applications. *Family Process, 18,* 3-28.

Patterson, J. M., & McCubbin, H. I. (1983). Chronic illness: Family stress and coping. In C. R. Figley & McCubbin (Eds.), *Stress and the family: Coping with catastrophe* (Vol. 2, pp. 21-36). New York: Brunner/Mazel.

Primomo, J., Yates, B. C., & Woods, N. F. (1990). Social support for women during chronic illness: The relationship among sources and types to adjustment. *Research in Nursing & Health, 13,* 153-161.

Robinson, J. P., Shaver, P. R., & Wrightsman, L. S. (1991). *Measures of personality and social psychological attitudes.* New York: Harcourt Brace Jovanovich.

Roosa, M. W., & Beals, J. (1990). Measurement issues in family assessment: The case of the Family Environment Scale. *Family Process, 29,* 191-198.

Smilkstein, G. (1978). The Family APGAR: A proposal for a family function test and its use by physicians. *Journal of Family Practice, 6*, 1231-1239.

Smilkstein, G., Ashworth, C., & Montana, D. (1982). Validity and reliability of the Family APGAR as a test of family function. *Journal of Family Practice, 15*, 303-311.

Spiegel, D., Bloom, J. R., & Gottheil, E. (1983). Family environment as a predictor of adjustment to metastatic breast carcinoma. *Journal of Psychosocial Oncology, 1*(1), 33-44.

Stetz, K. M., Lewis, F. M., & Primomo, J. (1986). Family coping strategies and chronic illness in the mother. *Family Relations, 28*, 515-522.

Vess, J. D., Moreland, J. R., & Schwebel, A. I. (1985). An empirical assessment of the effects of cancer on family role functioning. *Journal of Psychosocial Oncology, 3*(1), 1-6.

Walker, L. S., McLaughlin, F. J., & Greene, J. W. (1988). Functional illness and family functioning: A comparison of healthy and somatizing adolescents. *Family Process, 27*, 317-325.

Wellisch, D. K., Gritz, E. R., Scahin, W., Wang, H. J., & Siau, J. (1991a). Psychological functioning of daughters of breast cancer patients. Part I. Daughters and comparison subjects. *Psychosomatics, 32*, 324-336.

Wellisch, D. K., Gritz, E. R., Scahin, W., Wang, H. J., & Siau, J. (1991b). Psychological functioning of daughters of breast cancer patients. Part II. Characterizing the distressed daughter of the breast cancer patient. *Psychosomatics, 33*, 171-179.

Woods, N. F., Haberman, M. R., & Packard, N. J. (1993). Demands of illness and individual, dyadic, and family adaptation in chronic illness. *Western Journal of Nursing Research, 15*(1), 10-30.

Zabora, J. R., & Smith, E. D. (1991). Family dysfunction and the cancer patient: Early recognition and intervention. *Oncology, 5*(2), 31-35.

Zabora, J. R., Smith, E. D., & Baker, F. (1993, October 2-4). Quality of life issues for families following bone marrow transplantation. Paper delivered during "Psycho-oncology V: Psychosocial Factors in Cancer Risk and Survival," New York, NY.

Zabora, J. R., Fetting, J. H., Shanley, V. B., Seddon, C. F., & Enterline, J. P. (1989). Predicting conflict with staff among families of cancer patients during prolonged hospitalizations. *Journal of Psychosocial Oncology, 7*(3), 103-111.

Zabora, J. R., Smith E. D., Baker, F., Wingard, J. R., & Curbow, B. (1992). The family: The other side of bone marrow transplantation. *Journal of Psychosocial Oncology, 10*(1), 35-46.

Commentary

David Spiegel, MD

This volume addresses the relationship between psychological, social, and spiritual resources and adjustment to cancer. The five well-written and thoughtful articles clearly indicate that these domains are important to understanding and improving adjustment to cancer and that all three domains are deeply interrelated and should be even more so. Religion, after all, is not merely an individual experience of faith but a social phenomenon, and religious practice mobilizes social support, especially at times of major life crises. Similarly, as noted, social support may influence coping style, shifting the focus from an uncontrollable primary problem such as advancing cancer to a controllable one such as influencing the effects of cancer, some of which are, of course, social and psychological.

The field is clearly moving toward a recognition that the ecological validity of the phenomena we study is crucial. The literature on coping has shown that there is no useful disposition to coping per se. Rather, the style of coping with a given stressor may influence a given outcome. We are moving from the study of traits to states, from general dispositions to specific outcomes. Thus, Suzanne Thompson and Mary Collins have usefully described the progres-

---

Dr. Spiegel is Professor, Department of Psychiatry and Behavioral Sciences, Stanford University School of Medicine, Stanford, CA 94305-5544.

[Haworth co-indexing entry note]: "Commentary." Spiegel, David. Co-published simultaneously in the *Journal of Psychosocial Oncology* (The Haworth Medical Press, an imprint of The Haworth Press, Inc.) Vol. 13, No. 1/2, 1995, pp. 115-121; and: *Psychosocial Resource Variables in Cancer Studies: Conceptual and Measurement Issues* (ed: Barbara Curbow, and Mark R. Somerfield), The Haworth Medical Press, an imprint of The Haworth Press, Inc., 1995, pp. 115-121. Multiple copies of this article/chapter may be purchased from The Haworth Document Delivery Center [1-800-3-HAWORTH; 9:00 a.m. - 5:00 p.m. (EST)]. *[Single or multiple copies of this article are available from The Haworth Document Delivery Service: 1-800-342-9678, 9:00 a.m. - 5:00 p.m. (EST)].*

115

sion from Rotter's important initial contribution (1975) of locus of control through Seligman's general model (1975) of learned helplessness to Bandura's specific self-efficacy theory (1982). The literature on locus of control has been divided into domains. One can perceive internal control in one but not another. Similarly, learned helplessness may not always generalize to all situations. Bandura found that self-efficacy is a concept that must be studied in specific contexts. This specificity of intrapsychic constructs nicely parallels the observation that patients facilitate adaptation by being flexible in their domains of control. Even though patients do not control the disease, they can control its effects on their lives or on the course of their treatment.

Michael Parle and Peter Maguire have provided a sensible and thoughtful overview of the applications of coping theory in the study of adjustment to cancer. They pointed out that early theories of coping emphasized behavior too much at the expense of cognition, but the introduction of the importance of appraisal tends to make the situation more important and the concept of coping more situation specific: a state more than a trait. As these authors noted, this necessary diversity of situations and responses makes comparison within and across scales more complex. They concluded that appraisal factors–e.g., hopelessness or pessimism–seem to be better related to adjustment than to any of a variety of behavioral coping strategies.

Parle and Maguire's recommendation that coping should be studied more in relation to mental health and physical outcome is an important one. These authors have appropriately emphasized Bandura's important concept of self-efficacy. This domain expands the concept of appraisal from that of the stressor to that of the person responding to the stressor, calling for an assessment of match between the demands of the situation and the person's abilities to respond to it. Sensibly, the authors have also called for a broader and more comprehensive assessment of the problems facing cancer patients: the illness and its treatment; the psychological domains of anxiety about the illness, self-esteem, and relationships; and the practical domains of work, finances, and day-to-day abilities.

Unfortunately, coping has been studied in individual isolation. The interaction between social support and coping has received far less attention; yet studies of group intervention, for example, suggest that coping styles can be powerfully influenced by social support (Spiegel, Bloom, & Yalom, 1981; Stein, Hermanson, & Spiegel, 1993). This sense of commonality of the ability to give as well as receive support that occurs in groups would naturally influence self-appraisal regarding the efficacy of coping, would expand and modify individuals' views of the threats facing them, would provide encouragement for more active coping, and would provide alternative models for coping strategies (Spiegel, 1993a). Similarly, belief systems, religious and otherwise, provide not only social connection but also alternative means of appraisal. An illness that is a meaningless tragedy in one context may acquire a different meaning in a group, a means of providing support to someone else in the same situation, or in a religious context, a means of testing faith. Thus, a systematic understanding of coping–ranging from appraisal of the illness as a stressor and self-efficacy to behavior–must include the individual, social, and cognitive environment as well.

The article on social support by Christina Blanchard and her colleagues provides a useful typology of mechanisms in social support involving cognitive components such as reappraisal and behavioral components such as adaptive counterresponses. They have underscored the fact that, in various ways, social support may reinforce control, but they do not emphasize enough the fact that the absence of social support amplifies anxiety–especially anxiety regarding death, isolation being a metaphor for death. The relationship between social isolation and death is not merely symbolic. It also is clear that social isolation is associated with an elevated risk of mortality from all causes (House, Landis, & Umberson, 1988) and specifically from cancer (Goodwin et al., 1987; Reynolds & Kaplan, 1990). Blanchard et al. are appropriately cautious about the literature linking social support and enhanced survival. However, their comments on our study showing that metastatic breast cancer patients randomly assigned to weekly support groups for a year live an average of 18 months longer than control patients do (Spiegel et al., 1989) imply that the absence of data on the patients' medical treatment after the beginning of the group intervention mitigates that finding. However, this is unlikely, first, because medical treatment for metastatic breast cancer is essentially palliative. The modem era of chemotherapy and radiation has extended survival time for three or four months at most. One irony of modern chemotherapy is that demonstrably reducing the tumor burden seems to have little effect on survival time. Second, we will soon publish new data demonstrating that subsequent medical treatment received by treatment and control groups in our study was similar.

The role of health care providers is one that clearly needs further research. It is disturbing to read that only 18 percent of cancer patients view health care providers as important members of their social support network despite frequent contact with providers. Yet the literature shows that patients want emotional support, not merely instrumental or informational support, from their physicians. This constitutes cognitive flexibility on the patients' part. Patients would like their physicians to give them primary control: that is, cure them of their disease. But their goals shift when they learn that is not possible. At that point, they want care instead of cure. I have routinely seen tears in the eyes of breast cancer patients when they describe what it meant to them when their oncologist gave them a hug, took their hand, or told them that no matter what happens, "I'll be there to help you." When cure is impossible, care is essential. This kind of social support enhances patients' sense of being in control of their treatment and their social environment, if not of their disease. When cure is impossible, care is essential.

Social support, whether instrumental or emotional, also may, in turn, influence spiritual factors, not only through the reinforcing effect of practicing a shared belief system, but in living it as well. In a much deeper sense, however, social support may allay spiritual concerns, or at least modify them. Cancer mobilizes a stark confrontation with mortality, a concept that is difficult to comprehend. One typical way in which we attempt to understand the concept is the sense of being alone. Isolation is thus a social and psychological metaphor for death. In the words of the old African-American spiritual, "You've got to walk that lonesome valley by yourself." Thus, anything that isolates someone socially will tend to reinforce death anxiety. Intense social involvement at a time of stress can therefore reduce the sense of the imminence of death, not through denying death, but rather through keeping it at bay. In addition, social support provides lessons about an array of coping styles ranging from techniques for modifying the

impact of chemotherapy to means of enhancing control over relationships and life goals, expanding the network of social involvement. This
expanded array of involvement provides alternative models for secondary control ranging from reducing the effects of the disease and
treatment to defining new goals that can be achieved in limited time.
Indeed, this can be a positive outcome of a life-threatening event
(Spiegel, 1993b; Spiegel, Bloom, & Yalom, 1981; Yalom & Greaves,
1977). That many cancer patients define the disease as having ironi-
cally positive aspects is no accident; what is important in life is uncovered and clarified. Time spent with family and friends takes on new
meaning when the time to do so is clearly limited.

Most investigators approach the subject of religious faith with
some temerity, as Richard Jenkins and Kenneth Pargament have
noted in their article. Religious faith, by its very nature, seems to
defy reduction to measurable variables. Yet these authors have done
an artful job of discussing types and proponents of religious faith.
Without attempting to explain religion in purely psychological or
social terms, religion, through imparting a system of meaning, is
indeed likely to help people restructure their experience of illness–to see it in a broader context, which may help them accept
what appears to be a meaningless tragedy as having meaning. There
may be other ways of accomplishing this: for example, by using the
illness as an occasion to give help to as well as receive help from
other people in a similar situation in a support group (Riessman,
1965; Spiegel, 1993b). Religious practice provides alternative
opportunities for doing this. It may help the ill person to accept
helplessness–the type of faith that puts the outcome in God's hands,
or to experience control by a restructured meaning, see suffering as
a test of faith or as a challenge to impart beliefs to others. It is easy
to dismiss some of the social components of religious faith, such as
"using" religion to elevate one's social standing or contacts rather
than "living" it. At the same time, just as religious faith may
influence cognition through restructuring the meaning of illness, it
also may extend the domain of social support by activating
resources that provide similar effects on cognition and behavior.

Patricia Fobair and James Zabora have provided a thoughtful
review of the major measures of family environment used to help
investigators address the related questions of how family environ-

ment influences patients' adjustment and vice versa. Certain measures, they conclude, work better as independent variables, whereas others work better as dependent variables. The Family Environment Scale (Moos, 1974) and the F-COPES (McCubbin, Larsen, & Olson, 1987) are used primarily as independent variables that predict subsequent adjustment. For example, more expressiveness and an atmosphere of open and shared problem solving in the families of metastatic breast cancer patients predict subsequent lower mood disturbance on the Profile of Mood States (Spiegel, Bloom, & Gottheil, 1983). These kinds of studies demonstrate specific ways in which the nature of the family environment can influence patients' adjustment. The FACES III has been used more as a dependent variable, demonstrating how illness or intervention can change the family environment. Both types of information are valuable because they demonstrate the impact of illness on families and the impact of families on illness. This line of research also underscores an important deficit in much of Western medicine: an emphasis on the individual as patient, with little attention paid to the impact of disease on the family. This failure is all the more crucial in an era when efforts at cost containment have placed far more of the caregiving burden on family members than ever before. Cancer constitutes not only a threat to the patient but also signals a rearrangement of caretaking roles in the family and the introduction of new needs and anxieties within the family. The emerging literature suggests that there are better and worse ways to deal with these challenges—that open and shared problem solving, expressiveness, intense mutual support, cohesion, and reduction of conflict facilitate the family's and patient's adaptation to illness.

The five articles have provided a thoughtful and useful review of the intrapsychic, interpersonal, and religious domains as they affect adjustment to cancer. They make a strong case that all three domains provide opportunities for understanding and improving patients' adjustment to life-threatening illness. These domains may influence biological as well as psychological and social processes. This is surprising only from a Cartesian perspective. Humans are social and psychological as well as biological creatures; we are shaped by our health and social environment in a causal sense. But we also define our environments through our attempts to create and restructure meaning in them. These efforts are especially important when disease changes one's physical, psychological, and social world. All of these domains are profoundly affected by illnesses such as cancer; yet they are clearly interacting resources that can be tapped adaptively in living well, even with a life-threatening illness.

REFERENCES

Bandura, A. (1982). The self and mechanisms in human agency. *American Psychologist, 37*, 122-147.

Goodwin, J. S., Hunt, W. C., Key, C. R., & Samet, J. M. (1987). The effect of marital status on stage, treatment and survival of cancer patients. *Journal of the American Medical Association, 158*, 3125-3130.

House, J. S., Landis, K. R., & Umberson, D. (1988). Social relationships and health. *Science, 241*, 540-544.

McCubbin, H. I., Larsen, A., & Olson, D. H. (1987). F-COPES: Family Crisis Oriented Personal Scales. In McCubbin & A. Thompson (Eds.), *Family assessment inventories for research and practice* Madison, WI:

Moos, R. (1974). *Family Environmental Scales.* Palo Alto, CA: Consulting Psychologists Press.

Reynolds, P., & Kaplan, G. (1990, Fall). Social connections and risk for cancer: Prospective evidence from the Alameda County Study. *Behavioral Medicine,* 101-110.

Riessman, F. (1965). The "helper therapy" principle. *Social Work, 10*, 27-32.

Rotter, J. B. (1975). Some problems and misconceptions related to the construct of internal vs. external control of reinforcement. *Journal of Consulting & Clinical Psychology, 48*, 56-67.

Seligman, M. (1975). *Helplessness: On Depression, Development, and Death.* San Francisco: Freeman.

Spiegel, D. (1993a). *Living beyond limits: New hope and help for facing life-threatening illness.* New York: Times Books.

Spiegel, D. (1993b). Psychosocial intervention in cancer. *Journal of the National Cancer Institute, 85*, 1198-1205.

Spiegel, D., Bloom, J. R., & Gottheil, E. (1983). Family environment of patients with metastatic carcinoma. *Journal of Psychosocial Oncology, 1*(1), 33-44.

Spiegel, D., Bloom, J. R., & Yalom, I. D. (1981). Group support for patients with metastatic breast cancer. *Archives of General Psychiatry, 38*, 527-533.

Spiegel, D., Bloom, J. R., Kraemer, H. C., & Gottheil, E. (1989, October 14). Effect of psychosocial treatment on survival of patients with metastatic breast cancer. *Lancet, ii*, 888-891.

Stein, S., Hermanson, K., & Spiegel, D. (1993). New directions in psycho-oncology. *Current Opinion in Psychiatry, 6*, 838-846.

Yalom, I., & Greaves, C. (1997). Group therapy with the terminally ill. *American Journal of Psychiatry, 134*, 396-400.

Assessment of Psychological Functioning in Cancer Patients

Carolyn Cook Gotay, PhD

Jeffrey D. Stern, MA

SUMMARY. This article identifies frequently used instruments that have been used to measure psychological functioning in cancer patients, summarizes information about the use of these tools in samples of cancer patients, and provides a critical evaluation of and recommendations for developing assessment instruments. Issues of the *Journal of Psychosocial Oncology* published between 1986 and 1993 were reviewed to select the scales most commonly used to measure patients' psychological functioning. Seven scales that assess depression, anxiety, psychological symptoms, mood, and general psychosocial adjustment to illness were identified: Beck Depression Inventory, Center for Epidemiological Studies-Depression, State-Trait Anxiety Inventory, Symptom Checklist 90-R, Brief Symptom Inventory, Profile of Mood States, and Psychosocial Adjustment to Illness Scale. A review of studies using the different scales in samples of cancer patients highlighted numerous issues concerning the validity of these tools. Future studies should address the following: psychometric evaluation as part of study

Dr. Gotay is an Associate Researcher and Mr. Stern is a Graduate Research Assistant, Cancer Research Center of Hawaii, Honolulu. (Address correspondence to Dr. Gotay, Cancer Research Center of Hawaii, 1236 Lauhala Street, Honolulu, HI 96813.) The authors wish to express their appreciation to Stephen B. Haynes, PhD, and the editors of this volume. Preparation of the article was supported in part by grants CA 61711 and CA 01642 from the National Cancer Institute.

[Haworth co-indexing entry note]: "Assessment of Psychological Functioning in Cancer Patients." Gotay, Carolyn Cook, and Jeffrey D. Stern. Co-published simultaneously in the *Journal of Psychosocial Oncology* (The Haworth Medical Press, an imprint of The Haworth Press, Inc.) Vol. 13, No. 1/2, 1995, pp. 123-160; and: *Psychosocial Resource Variables in Cancer Studies: Conceptual and Measurement Issues* (ed: Barbara Curbow, and Mark R. Somerfield), The Haworth Medical Press, an imprint of The Haworth Press, Inc., 1995, pp. 123-160. *[Single or multiple copies of this article are available from The Haworth Document Delivery Service: 1-800-342-9678, 9:00 a.m. - 5:00 p.m. (EST)].*

designs, content validation in cancer patients, reduction of items, study samples, the use of norms, interpretation of scale scores, and inclusion of information in addition to self-reports whenever possible. *[Article are available from The Haworth Document Delivery Service: 1-800-342-9678.]*

Measurement is central to psychosocial oncology. Psychosocial research may seek to describe cancer patients' well-being, evaluate the impact of an intervention, or (as the articles in this volume encourage) investigate the role of resource variables on patients' well-being. Regardless, the ultimate value of the research rests on its use of sound assessment instruments. The first questions raised when designing a study often include "What scales should I use?" closely followed by "Have these instruments been used previously with cancer patients? Are they reliable and valid?" These questions are often difficult to answer because of the wide diversity of publications where psychosocial oncology research appears.

Relatively early in the short history of psychosocial oncology, measurement was a central focus, as reflected in the American Cancer Society's first workshop on psychosocial oncology in 1983, which focused extensively on assessment issues (ACS, 1984). A number of papers presented at that meeting identified available instruments and made recommendations for their use with cancer patients. Since that time, selected instruments such as the Profile of Mood States (POMS) and the Rosenberg Self-Esteem Scale have been critically evaluated (e.g., Cella et al., 1987; Curbow & Somerfield, 1991; Guadagnoli & Mor, 1989). Less attention, however, has been focused on general issues in assessment, on tools that are commonly used in cancer patient populations, and on comparisons of different instruments.

This article (1) identifies and reviews tools that have often been used to measure cancer patients' psychological functioning, (2) summarizes information about how these tools are used in these populations, and (3) provides a critical evaluation of and recommendations for developing assessment instruments. We focus on psychological functioning in adults: that is, outcomes that emphasize an individual's adjustment to cancer. Many terms have been used to denote psychological functioning, including emotional well-being, mood, happiness, coping, adjustment, distress, psychosocial problems, and psychiatric morbidity. This review includes instruments that measure several specific aspects of psychological functioning: depression, anxiety, psychological symptoms, mood, and general psychological adjustment to illness.

Issues related to cancer patients' quality of life have received considerable attention in recent years (e.g., Tchekmedyian & Cella, 1990; Nayfield, Hailey, & McCabe, 1990), including the development of a number of assessment scales (cf. Cella & Tulsky, 1990). Although most quality-of-life scales include a psychological component as part of a multidimensional assessment of overall quality of life, they do not provide detailed information about psychological well-being per se. To limit our focus to overall psychological well-being, we excluded outcomes related to specific domains of functioning such as treatment-related symptoms, activities of daily living, social and family functioning, body image, and sexual functioning. Measurement issues in some of these areas have been discussed (e.g., Cull, 1992; Hopwood, 1993), whereas others remain to be examined in the future.

METHOD

Identification of Instruments

We identified the instruments used to measure psychological functioning by reviewing all issues of the *Journal of Psychosocial Oncology* published between 1986 and mid-1993. The task was limited to articles that included (1) at least one measure of psychological functioning, excluding multidimensional quality of life, (2) data collection (no reviews), (3) adult patients rather than families, health care providers, or healthy populations, (4) self-report instruments, and (5) scales with reported validity and reliability (either in the *Journal of Psychosocial Oncology* or elsewhere).

Thirty issues of the journal were reviewed, and 41 articles met our inclusion criteria. More than 40 different instruments of psychological functioning were used in these studies; many were discussed in only one report. (A complete list of the scales is available from the first author.) When we tabulated the number of times each scale was used, the results were the seven scales listed in Table 1.

TABLE 1. Scales of Psychological Adjustment.

Scale	Number of Items	Scores Available
Beck Depression Inventory (BDI)	21	Depression
Center for Epidemiological Studies-Depression (CES-D)	20	Depression
State-Trait Anxiety Inventory (STAI)	40	State Anxiety, Trait Anxiety
Symptom Checklist 90-R (SCL-90-R)	90	Global: Global Severity Scores, Positive Symptoms Distress Index, Postitive Symptom Total. Dimensions: Somatization, Depression, Psychoticism, Anxiety, Obsessive-Compulsive, Phobic Anxiety, Hostility, Interpersonal Sensitivity, Paranoid Ideation
Brief Symptom Inventory (BSI)	53	Same as the SCL-90-R
Profile of Mood States (POMS)	65	Total: Total Mood Disturbance. Subscales: Tension-Anxiety, Depression-Dejection, Anger-Hostility, Vigor-Activity, Fatigue-Inertia, Confusion-Bewilderment
Psychosocial Adjustment to Illness Scale–Self-Report (PAIS-SR)	46	Factors: Health Care Orientation, Vocational Environment, Domestic Environment, Sexual Relationships, Extended Family Relationships, Social Environment, Psychological Distress

All other scales were used in no more than two studies, with the exception of the Locke-Wallace Scale of Marital Adjustment (Locke & Wallace, 1959), which was used in five studies. Because the Locke-Wallace scale focuses specifically on one relationship, it is not included here; however, investigators may wish to note its fairly heavy use with cancer patients.

We sought additional information about the use of the seven scales in other psychosocial oncology literature and reviewed information about their original development and validation. A Medline search of the cancer literature available in English was conducted for the same time period using the names of the instruments to identify additional studies in which the scales had been used. This search was augmented further by reviewing lists of references and searching additional journals by hand. Although we are aware that references found with these strategies do not represent an exhaustive list, we believe that a representative sample of the available literature was reviewed.

Scales of Psychological Functioning

As summarized in Table 1, the Beck Depression Inventory (BDI) and Center for Epidemiological Studies-Depression scale (CES-D) assess depression, the State-Trait Anxiety Inventory (STAI) assesses anxiety, the Symptom Checklist-90-Revised (SCL-90-R) and the Brief Symptom Inventory (BSI) assess psychological symptoms, the POMS assesses mood, and the Psychological Adjustment to Illness Scale-Self-Report (PAIS-SR) assesses general psychological adjustment to illness. All these scales are relatively brief (taking 30 minutes or less to complete, with most estimated to take 15 minutes or less), and the majority include subscale scores as well as a total score. Because most of these scales are copyrighted, investigators must obtain permission and pay a per-administration fee to use them. Many copyright holders offer test manuals with extensive information about the scale, including instructions for administration, and services for computer-assisted scoring of the tests. None of the scales was developed specifically for cancer patients. Most have been used widely in noncancer patient populations, especially in psychiatric samples (Bech, 1992; Rabkin & Klein, 1987) and in samples with other medical conditions (Derogatis & Wise, 1989).

Each scale is described briefly, with special attention to how it was originally validated. Findings of studies that have used each scale with cancer patients are reviewed in Table 2, which is designed to serve as a resource for readers, who can add additional studies to the table. In the text, overall themes in the findings are summarized when possible, although the large variability in patient populations and study designs prevent drawing definitive conclusions.

TABLE 2. Selected Studies on the Psychological Functioning of Cancer Patients (1986-93): Measures Used, Patient Populations, and Key Findings.

Beck Depression Inventory (BDI)

Bisno & Richardson, 1987. *Subjects:* 53 patients newly diagnosed with mixed cancers receiving radiation therapy. *Findings:* No difference in depression scores by cancer site, ethnicity, or employment status. Scores of 70% were in the normal range (0-13), 21% were moderately depressed, and 2% were severely depressed.

Carpenter, Morrow, & Schmale, 1989. *Subjects:* 43 patients diagnosed with early Hodgkin's disease. Half completed treatment less than 2 years before the study, and half completed it more than 2 years before. *Findings:* No significant differences in depression scores between the two groups.

Heim & Oei, 1993. *Subjects:* 47 patients with or without pain who had completed treatment for prostate cancer in various stages. *Findings:* Patients with pain scored significantly higher ($p < .05$) than those without pain.

Noyes et al., 1990. *Subjects:* 438 patients with mixed solid tumors (stage not reported). *Findings:* 86% were not depressed according to the psychological items.

Spiegel & Sands, 1988. *Subjects:* 62 patients with mixed cancers at different stages. Six Factorial design: 2 (high or low pain) × 3 (psychotherapy, pharmacotherapy, or hypnosis). *Findings:* The high-pain group scored significantly higher than did those in the little- or no-pain group. Findings confirmed earlier reports of a link between pain and mood disturbance in cancer patients.

Center for Epidemiological Studies–Depression Scale (CES-D)

Challis & Stam, 1992. *Subjects:* 70 patients with mixed cancers (stage not reported) who were tested before chemotherapy was initiated and before each of 6 chemotherapy sessions. *Findings:* Significantly greater depression was found at baseline than at chemotherapy sessions 2, 3, 4, and 6.

Edgar, Rosberger, & Nowlis, 1992. *Subjects:* 205 patients with various mixed-stage cancers who received a psychosocial intervention either at diagnosis or 4 months later. Testing was done at baseline and at 4, 8, and 12 months. *Findings:* Depression was reduced at 4 and 8 months after diagnosis and leveled off at 12 months. The intervention was more effective at 4 months after diagnosis than at diagnosis.

Fobair, Hoppe, & Bloom, 1986. *Subjects:* 403 survivors of mixed-stage Hodgkin's disease who were tested 1-21 years after treatment. *Findings:* 37% were not satisfied with their energy levels. Low energy correlated with depression.

Gritz, Wellisch, & Landsverk, 1988. *Subjects:* 88 patients with mixed-stage seminomatous or nonseminomatous testicular cancer who were tested before treatment and 6 months, 3 years, and 4 years after treatment. *Findings:* No between-group differences or variations were observed over time. However, nearly one-third of the patients had sought psychological help since their diagnosis.

Gritz et al., 1990. *Subjects:* 34 patients with mixed-stage testicular cancer and their wives tested 1-7.5 years after treatment. *Findings:* Scores for patients and wives were highly correlated and did not differ significantly from those in the standardization sample.

Roberts et al., 1990. *Subjects:* 100 patients with breast cancer (stage not reported) divided into 4 groups: survivors vs. controls and interviewed vs. not interviewed. Testing was done after treatment ended. *Findings:* Survivors had significantly higher scores than controls. No differences were found between the interview and no interview groups.

Stam, Koopmans, & Mathieson, 1991. *Subjects:* 51 laryngectomy patients tested after treatment. *Findings:* A lower aggregated "distress" score was predicted best by two variables: the physician met the patient's needs and a laryngectomee visited the patient before surgery.

State-Trait Anxiety Inventory (STAI)

Carpenter, Morrow, & Schmale, 1989. *Subjects:* See BDI. *Findings:* State anxiety did not differ as a function of time since treatment ended (less or more than 2 years before).

Challis & Stam, 1992. *Subjects:* See CES-D. *Findings:* Patients with anticipatory nausea and vomiting reported significantly greater state anxiety than did other patients, a difference that persisted through the 6 weekly sessions.

Haut et al., 1991. *Subjects:* 36 patients with mixed cancers (stage not reported) who were tested in a timed series while receiving chemotherapy. *Findings:* State anxiety did not differ between patients who did or did not experience nausea and vomiting after treatment ended.

Heim & Oei, 1993. *Subjects:* See BDI. *Findings:* Patients without pain had less state anxiety than did those with pain.

Hursti et al., 1992. *Subjects:* 39 patients with testicular cancer (stage not reported) who were tested 1-6 years after chemotherapy. *Findings:* In part, trait anxiety mediated the persistence or extinction of conditioned nausea.

TABLE 2. (continued)

Leinster et al., 1989. *Subjects:* 59 patients with early stage breast cancer who were tested before and 3 and 12 months after surgery. *Findings:* Mean scores approximated those for general surgical patients and did not indicate pathology. A high concern about appearance and uncertainty about the diagnosis were associated with higher anxiety.

Morrow, 1992. *Subjects:* 299 patients with various cancers in mixed stages who were tested during chemotherapy. *Findings:* Anxiety was associated with development of anticipatory nausea and vomiting ($p < .05$).

Spiegel & Sands, 1988. *Subjects:* See BDI. *Findings:* The high-pain group scored significantly higher than the low-pain group on items assessing fright and worry and significantly lower on items assessing relaxation and feeling steady ($p < .05$).

Stam, Koopmans, & Mathieson, 1991. *Subjects:* See CES-D. *Findings:* Anxiety-related problems were associated with length of hospitalization after laryngectomy, inadequate social support, and postsurgical life-style changes.

Wong & Bramwell, 1992. *Subjects:* 25 breast cancer patients with mixed-stage breast cancer who were tested 1-2 days before hospital discharge and 1-2 weeks after discharge. *Findings:* No change in state anxiety occurred between the 2 time periods; at both times, state anxiety scores were significantly elevated compared with normals.

Symptom Checklist 90-Revised (SCL-90-R)

Bruera et al., 1989. *Subjects:* 64 patients receiving treatment for advanced breast cancer. *Findings:* Psychological distress correlated with asthenia.

Carter, Carter, & Siliunas, 1993. *Subjects:* 28 patients with Stage I or II breast cancer and their husbands tested 2-3 years after mastectomy. *Findings:* Neither patients' nor spouses' scores were significantly elevated and were not significantly different.

Hannum et al., 1991. *Subjects:* 22 patients with Stage I or II breast cancer and their husbands who were tested 9-12 months after diagnosis. *Findings:* Spouses' coping behaviors and ratings of their marital relationship were the best predictors of patients' psychological distress.

Heinrich & Schag, 1987. *Subjects:* 57 veterans with mixed cancers at various stages and healthy veterans (testing sequence not reported). *Findings:* Patients scored higher than controls on the Depression and Global Severity subscales but not on the Anxiety subscale. Only the patients' depression scores were significantly elevated above normal ($T > 60$).

Irwin & Kramer, 1988. *Subjects:* 181 male and female patients treated with radiation for mixed cancers (stage not reported) who were interviewed at the onset of treatment, 1 week later, and 2 months after treatment ended. *Findings:* Social and socioemotional support were only moderately associated with reduced psychological distress after treatment. Sustained support was not predictive of amelioration of distress.

Irwin et al., 1986. *Subjects:* See Irwin & Kramer, 1988. *Findings:* Patients reported significantly less depression and anxiety after treatment, but their subscale scores remained elevated at 2 months posttreatment. No sex differences were identified.

Johnstone et al., 1991. *Subjects:* 70 patients with mixed-stage testicular cancer and 38 with mixed stage Hodgkin's disease who were tested before and after treatment. *Findings:* Outpatients with testicular cancer showed no significant improvement from significantly elevated scores on 8 subscales, whereas outpatients with Hodgkin's improved on 6 of 7 subscales.

Morrow, 1992. *Subjects:* See STAI. *Findings:* Anxiety scores were associated with development of anticipatory nausea and vomiting ($p < .05$).

Quinn, Fontana, & Reznikoff, 1986. *Subjects:* 60 male patients with mixed-stage lung cancer and their wives who were tested 1 month after diagnosis and 44 couples again 3 months later. *Findings:* Support was related to distress as well as change in distress. Patients and spouses who used wish-fulfilling fantasy to cope experienced unabating psychological distress; those who used cognitive restructuring and information seeking were less distressed.

Roberts et al., 1992. *Subjects:* 32 survivors of gynecologic cancer (stage not reported) for more than 1 year who were tested 1-19 years after surgery. *Findings:* The patients scored at least 1 standard deviation above the mean on the Somatization, Obsessive Compulsiveness, Depression, Phobic Anxiety, and Psychoticism subscales.

Silverman-Dresner & Restaino-Baumann, 1990-91. *Subjects:* 374 women divided into 4 groups: breast cancer patients self-help, reconstructed, no aftercare, and healthy women. *Findings:* No significant differences were found in the scores between groups. (See, also, Silverman-Dresner, 1989-90; Silverman-Dressner & Restaino-Baumann, 1989.)

Brief Symptom Inventory (BSI)

Baider & Kaplan De-Nour, 1986. *Subjects:* 30 Moslem or Jewish women with mixed-stage breast cancer who had completed treatment. *Findings:* Moslem women scored higher on all subscales except anxiety.

TABLE 2 (continued)

Baider, Peretz, & Kaplan De-Nour, 1989. *Subjects:* 78 male and female patients with mixed-stage colon cancer who had completed treatment and their spouses. *Findings:* Males were less distressed than females. Wives of male patients were less distressed than husbands of female patients.

Baider, Peretz, & Kaplan De-Nour, 1992. *Subjects:* 106 male and female patients with mixed cancers at various stages who had completed treatment. Half were Holocaust survivors; the other half were matched with survivors for demographic and disease characteristics. *Findings:* Psychological distress was significantly greater in Holocaust survivors. Most subscale differences were significant at $p < .10$. No significant differences by sex were found.

Bloom et al., 1987. *Subjects:* 145 women with Stage I or II breast cancer treated by mastectomy, 90 with gall bladder disease treated by cholecystectomy, 87 with benign breast tumors who had biopsies, and 90 healthy women. All were tested 3, 6, 9, and 12 months after treatment ended. *Findings:* Mastectomy patients had consistently higher scores over time than did the comparison groups on the somatic distress factor only.

Cassileth et al., 1989. *Subjects:* 128 recently diagnosed patients with mixed cancers at various stages who were tested immediately after diagnosis and 6 and 12 months later. *Findings:* Satisfaction with care was independent of emotional status. Mood disturbance and psychological symptomatology were highly correlated. Emotional status improved with time.

Gilbar, 1991. *Subjects:* 140 patients who completed chemotherapy for mixed cancers (stage not reported) refused or dropped out of chemotherapy. *Findings:* Patients who dropped out of treatment scored significantly higher on the Obsessive-Complusive, Psychoticism, and Hostility subscales ($p < .05$). (See, also, Gilbar, 1989; Gilbar & De-Nour, 1988.)

Gilbar & Florian, 1991. *Subjects:* 60 patients with operable or inoperable mixed-stage breast cancer tested before their final treatment. *Findings:* Women with inoperable cancer scored higher than a group matched in age and time of diagnosis on the Somatization, Depression, Hostility, and Psychoticism subscales.

Kornblith et al., 1992a. *Subjects:* 273 male and female survivors of advanced-stage Hodgkin's disease tested 1-20 years ($M = 6.3$ years) after treatment. *Findings:* Psychological distress of both males and females averaged one standard deviation above the mean for healthy individuals ($T > 60$).

Kornblith et al., 1992b. *Subjects:* 93 survivors of advanced Hodgkin's disease treated with MOPP, ABVD, or both who were tested 1-20 years after treatment. *Findings:* No difference in distress according to chemotherapy regimen.

Northouse, 1988. *Subjects:* 50 newly diagnosed patients with mixed-stage breast cancer and their husbands who were tested 3 and 30 days after surgery. *Findings:* Psychosocial adjustment was related to patients' and husbands' levels of social support at both testing periods.

Northouse & Swain, 1987. *Subjects:* See Northouse, 1988. *Findings:* Levels of distress were significantly elevated in patients and husbands compared with the general population. General parity between patients' and husbands' distress, which did not improve across time.

Oberst & Scott, 1988. *Subjects:* 40 patients with bowel or urinary cancer (stage not reported) treated with surgery and their spouses who were tested before discharge and 10, 30, 60, and 120 days afterward. *Findings:* The intensity of distress was similar for patients and spouses. Patients' distress peaked 10 days after discharge, whereas spouses' distress peaked before discharge.

Sneed, Edlund, & Dias, 1992. *Subjects:* Male and female patients with various mixed-stage cancers who were divided into three groups: men, women with breast or gynecologic cancer, and women with other cancers. Testing was done 2 to 30 days after diagnosis. *Findings:* No sex differences in scores were found. Women with gynecologic or breast cancer were significantly less depressed, anxious, and hostile than were women with other types of cancer.

Syrjala, Cummings, & Donaldson, 1992. *Subjects:* 67 patients with hematologic cancers treated with bone marrow transplantation (BMT) and divided into four groups: usual care, therapist control, cognitive behavioral, hypnosis. Testing occurred before and after BMT. *Findings:* Scores used as a pre-BMT covariate strongly predicted nausea but did not predict vomiting during BMT.

Profile of Mood States (POMS)

Bloom et al., 1988. *Subjects:* 85 survivors of mixed-stage Hodgkin's disease who were tested after treatment ended. *Findings:* Change in leisure activities was the only significant predictor of mood distress ($p < .05$).

Cassileth et al., 1989. *Subjects:* See BSI. *Findings:* Mood disturbance was significantly lower at the second and third testings than at the first, indicating improvement in mood over time.

Cochran et al., 1987. *Subjects:* 36 patients with mixed-stage endometrial cancer and their husbands who were tested after treatment ended. *Findings:* Total scores were significantly correlated with sexual satisfaction even when pretreatment ratings and prognosis were controlled for. Data correlating spousal mood and changes in sexual behavior were not reported.

TABLE 2 (continued)

Edbril & Rieker, 1989. *Subjects:* 74 patients with testicular cancer (stages not reported) who were tested after treatment ended. *Findings:* Patients who reported less work satisfaction also reported significantly more tension-anxiety and depression-dejection than did a comparison group of patients who reported no change in work satisfaction.

Fawzy et al., 1990a, 1990b. *Subjects:* 62 melanoma patients with a good prognosis; half received a brief psychiatric intervention. Testing was done at baseline, after the intervention, and 6 months later. *Findings:* The intervention group had better outcomes after the intervention and to an even greater degree 6 months later. Scores correlated with coping styles and immunological measures.

Graydon, 1988. *Subjects:* 79 patients with breast or lung cancer (stages not reported) who were tested during treatment and 4-13 weeks afterward. *Findings:* After diagnosis and age, tension-anxiety scores were the best predictor of patients' functioning.

Gritz, Wellisch, & Landsverk, 1988. *Subjects:* See CES-D. *Findings:* Only the Fatigue-Inertia subscale differentiated the two groups. Scores were generally consistent with those from previous studies.

Gritz et al., 1990. *Subjects:* See CES-D. *Findings:* Scores were within the normal range for both patients and spouses.

Kornblith et al., 1992a. *Subjects:* See BSI. *Findings:* Psychological distress scores correlated with BSI scores.

Kornblith et al., 1992b. *Subjects:* See BSI. *Findings:* Psychosocial adjustment scores were predicted by infertility index and family income 1 month before the diagnosis.

Kukull, McCorkle, & Driever, 1986. *Subjects:* 53 patients with advanced lung cancer who were tested 1 or 2 months after diagnosis. *Findings:* Scores at both testing periods were not related to long-term survival ($ps > .10$).

Lerman et al., 1993. *Subjects:* 97 patients with Stage I or II breast cancer who were tested before and 3 months after mastectomy. *Findings:* Patients reporting difficulty communicating with the medical team reported more anxiety, depression, anger, and confusion at the 3-month follow-up.

Lichtman, Taylor, & Wood, 1987. *Subjects:* 78 patients with mixed-stage breast cancer (testing sequence not reported). *Findings:* Adjustment (determined by POMS total scores and 5 other measures) was better in patients who perceived greater social support from family members and friends.

Magid & Golomb, 1989. *Subjects:* 104 patients with mixed-stage leukemia who were employed or voluntarily or involuntarily unemployed and were tested during treatment. *Findings:* Those involuntarily unemployed had significantly higher depression and tension scores than the other groups.

Morrow, 1992. *Subiects:* See STAI. *Findings:* Anxiety was not associated with development of anticipatory nausea and vomiting ($p > .05$).

Pozo et al., 1992. *Subjects:* 63 patients with Stage I or II breast cancer who chose mastectomy or lumpectomy or had a mastectomy without any choice. Testing was done with abbreviated POMS subscales before and after surgery and 3, 6, and 12 months later. *Findings:* The surgical groups did not differ in distress or friendliness. A general trend across groups existed for distress to diminish with time.

Stam, Koopmans, & Mathieson, 1991. *Subjects:* See CES-D. *Findings:* Distress at follow-up was predicted best by current illness, dissatisfaction with social support, and life-style adjustment difficulties. (POMS short form and overall distress scores were used.)

Waligora-Serafin et al., 1992. *Subjects:* 44 newly diagnosed patients with mixed cancers in various stages who were assessed during treatment and 3 and 6 months after treatment ended. *Findings:* Mood disturbance was strongly associated with a number of psychosocial concerns (via Inventory of Current Concerns). Mood disturbance and number of concerns tapered off over time.

Psychosocial Adjustment to Illness Scale (PAIS)

Baider & Kaplan De-Nour, 1986. *Subjects:* See BSI. *Findings:* Moslem women had more adjustment problems. Differences were not significant because of high intersubject variability.

Baider, Peretz, & Kaplan De-Nour, 1989. *Subjects:* See BSI. *Findings:* Males were better adjusted than females, and wives of male patients were better adjusted than husbands of female patients.

Baider, Peretz, & Kaplan De-Nour, 1992. *Subjects:* See BSI. *Findings:* Holocaust survivors' adjustment to cancer tended to be poorer on 2 of 4 subscales: Health Care Orientation ($p < .10$) and Social Environment ($p < .08$).

Berckman & Austin, 1993. *Subjects:* 61 patients with mixed-stage lung cancer tested during outpatient treatment. *Findings:* Internal attributions for the cause of cancer were linked to significantly poorer adjustment, whereas perceived control was not.

Carter, Carter, & Siliunas, 1993. *Subjects:* See STAI. *Findings:* Neither patients nor spouses were psychologically symptomatic; both adjusted well to the mastectomy.

Cella, Mahon, & Donovan, 1990. *Subjects:* 40 patients with recurrent mixed cancers who were receiving treatment (testing sequence not reported). *Findings:* The patients were significantly more distressed than a normative group of cancer patients. *T* scores for health care orientation and psychological distress were notably high (*T*s > 70).

Durà & Ibañez, 1991. *Subjects:* 71 patients with mixed-stage breast cancer divided into three groups: controls, patients given information, patients and families given information. Testing was done before treatment and 1 and 5 months after treatment ended. *Findings:* Patients who received information were significantly better adjusted than the controls on most subscales. Group differences at 5 months indicated that additional information facilitated adjustment in a number of psychosocial areas.

Friedman et al., 1988a. *Subjects:* 57 patients with mixed-stage breast cancer divided into 4 groups on the basis of family cohesion. *Findings:* Patients in families with greater cohesion were better adjusted (*p* < .05). No significant relationship was found between adjustment and familial adaptability.

Friedman et al., 1988b. *Subjects:* 67 patients with mixed-stage breast cancer who were tested during treatment. *Findings:* Avoidant coping was related to poorer psychosocial adjustment, whereas active coping was associated with better adjustment on all subscales except health care orientation.

Friedman et al., 1990. *Subjects:* 49 patients with mixed-stage breast cancer. (Timing sequence of testing not reported.) *Findings:* Fighting spirit was related to better adjustment, whereas avoidant coping was related to poorer adjustment. Denial was unrelated to all adjustment measures.

Gilbar, 1991. *Subjects:* See BSI. *Findings:* Dropouts reported poorer adjustment than those who completed treatment on 5 of 7 domains (*p* < .05). (See, also, Gilbar, 1989; Gilbar & De-Nour, 1988.)

Gotcher, 1992. *Subjects:* 102 patients receiving treatment for various cancers (stages not reported). *Findings:* Communicating with significant others in an emotionally supportive environment was conducive to effective adjustment.

Greer et al., 1992. *Subjects:* 156 patients with advanced mixed cancers, 72 of whom were randomly assigned to receive psychotherapy. Testing was done before the intervention and 8 weeks and 4 months afterward. *Findings:* Patients who received psychotherapy showed greater improvement on most adjustment measures. This improvement increased over the course of follow-up.

Kornblith et al., 1992a. *Subjects:* See BSI. *Findings:* Developing a serious illness after cancer treatment ended was significantly related to poorer adaptation.

TABLE 2. (continued)

Kornblith et al., 1992b. *Subjects:* See BSI. *Findings:* No differences in psychosocial adaptation were found among Hodgkin's survivors exposed to different chemotherapy treatments.

Lowery, Jacobsen, & DuCette, 1993. *Subjects:* 195 patients with mixed-stage breast cancer who asked or did not ask "Why me?" Testing was done 1-60 months after diagnosis. *Findings:* Psychosocial adjustment improved as time since diagnosis increased. Higher mean total scores were related to "Why me?" thinking.

Northouse, 1988. *Subjects:* See BSI. *Findings:* Psychosocial and role adjustment was better in patients and husbands who received high levels of social support 3 and 30 days after treatment.

Northouse & Swain, 1987. *Subjects:* See BSI. *Findings:* Patients' total scores were significantly higher than their husbands'. Patients also reported significantly more role adjustment problems involving vocational, domestic, and social role domains than did husbands.

Next, information about the psychometric properties of the scales when used with cancer patients is reviewed. Of particular interest are *validity,* which refers to the ability of a scale to measure what it purports to assess; *content validity,* the extent to which the scale reflects all aspects of the construct being measured; *construct validity,* the degree to which it provides a sensitive and specific measure of the particular construct; and *criterion validity,* the degree to which it covaries with established measures of the construct. *Reliability* refers to the consistency of scale results over time (test-retest), the consistency of observers, and the consistency within the scale itself. (For additional discussions of psychometric issues, see Breckler, this volume, and Anastasi, 1988; DeVellis, 1991; Goldstein & Herson, 1990; Nunnally & Bernstein, 1994; Suen, 1990.)

OVERVIEW OF THE SELECTED SCALES

Beck Depression Inventory. The BDI (Beck et al., 1961) consists of 21 multiple-choice items related to symptoms of depression. Respondents rate their current feelings on a four-point scale of severity. Items are summed to yield a total depression score. The scale was originally developed for and validated on psychiatric patients, and its internal consistency as well as its sensitivity to clinician-rated changes in depression were supported. Beck and Beamesderfer (1974) recommended cutoffs both for screening depression in psychiatric patients and for research purposes. The BDI is among the most widely used self-report questionnaires in the literature, and a great deal of psychometric information is available. It was used in only a handful of studies reviewed here; however, overall, depression appears to be infrequent in cancer patients (Bisno & Richardson, 1987; Heim & Oei, 1993; Noyes et al., 1990), although pain increases the likelihood of depression (Heim & Oei, 1993; Spiegel & Sands, 1988).

Center for Epidemiological Studies-Depression. The CES-D (Weissman et al., 1977) was derived from other measures of depression, including the BDI. It contains 20 symptom-related items; respondents rate the frequency of having experienced these symptoms during the past week on four-point scales. Developed for use in both psychiatric and community samples, the scale distinguishes reliably among inpatient populations and is sensitive to changes over time. Interpretation of scores also is facilitated by a score cutoff point of 16, which reflects that 6 of 20 symptoms are at least moderately persistent. Scores above this cutoff are likely to indicate clinical depression in a full clinical evaluation. For the most part, depression assessed with the CES-D seems to improve in cancer patients over time (Challis & Stam, 1992; Edgar, Rosberger, & Nowlis, 1992), but not in all areas (Fobair, Hoppe, & Bloom, 1986; Gritz, Wellisch, & Landsverk, 1988) (see Table 2).

State-Trait Anxiety Inventory. The STAI (Spielberger, Gorsuch, & Lushene, 1970) consists of two scales of 20 items each: the State Anxiety Scale, which asks respondents to describe how they feel at a particular moment, and the Trait Anxiety Scale, which relates to how they generally feel. Respondents rate each item on a four-point scale. The STAI was developed on a large sample of high school and college students and demonstrated high levels of internal consistency and test-retest reliability. The independence of state from trait anxiety was supported in the original scale validation. Several studies investigated the STAI in relation to cancer-related symptoms. Anxiety (state, trait, or overall) was correlated with anticipatory nausea and vomiting and conditioned nausea (Challis & Stam, 1992; Hursti et al., 1992; Morrow, 1992), but not in all studies (Haut et al., 1991). Pain also was associated with higher STAI scores (Heim & Oei, 1993; Spiegel & Sands, 1988).

Symptom Checklist-90-Revised. The SCL-90 was developed to measure current psychological symptoms. Both interviewer-administered and self-administered (SCL-90-R) versions are available. As its name suggests, it consists of 90 items, which respondents endorse according to "how much discomfort that problem has been causing you during the past week." The SCL-90-R yields three indexes of general distress: the Global Severity Index (psychological distress), the Positive Symptom Distress Index (patient's style in experiencing distress), and the Positive Symptom Total (total number of symptoms reported). It also provides a measure of nine specific dimensions of psychological dysfunction. The SCL-90-R was validated in large groups of individuals, including psychiatric inpatients and outpatients, normal adults and adolescents, and cancer patients. As predicted, initial validation demonstrated strong internal consistency and test-retest reliability as well as concurrent validity with other, similar instruments. Several studies listed in Table 2 indicate elevated scores in cancer patients compared with normative groups on some subscales (Bruera et al., 1989; Heinrich & Schag, 1987; Roberts et al., 1992). Social support predicted less distress in one study (Quinn, Fontana, & Reznikoff, 1986) but not in another (Irwin & Kramer, 1988). No consistent subscale findings were found.

Brief Symptom Inventory. The BSI (Derogatis, 1975a, Derogatis & Melisaratos, 1983), the short version of the SCL-90-R, is considered separately here because both measures have been used extensively with cancer patients. The BSI consists of 53 items and yields three general scores and nine specific subscale scores per the longer version. The BSI has been validated in large samples of psychiatric in- and outpatients as well as in normative samples. It correlates highly on all SCL-90-R dimensions (all $rs > .92$). A variety of correlates of BSI scores were identified, each in a single study (see Table 2), with no consistent themes. Distress appeared to change little in the short term (Northouse & Swain, 1987). Although distress improved over a longer period (Cassileth et al., 1989), elevated distress was still seen in long-term cancer survivors (Kornblith et al., 1992). Studies that investigated sex differences found inconsistent results: Baider, Peretz, and Kaplan De-Nour (1989) found sex differences in both patients and spouses, whereas no such differences were found in several other studies (Northouse, 1988; Northouse & Swain, 1987; Oberst & Scott, 1988; Sneed, Edlund, & Dias, 1992).

Profile of Mood States. The POMS (McNair, Lorr, & Droppleman, 1971), designed to identify and assess transient and fluctuating affective states, consists of 65 adjectives describing feelings, which respondents rate for frequency of experiencing them over the past week on five-point scales. The instrument yields a total mood disturbance score as well as six factor scores. It was originally validated on psychiatric outpatients and normal controls. Its test-retest reliability was high, and it demonstrated sensitivity to emotional changes in patient groups. The POMS also has high concurrent validity with related scales. Several brief forms of the POMS have been developed for cancer patients (Cella et al., 1987; Guadagnoli & Mor, 1989; Shacham, 1983).

Despite heavy use of the POMS with cancer patients, few conclusions could be drawn on the basis of the results reported in Table 2, probably because of varying samples, different correlates, and so forth. Total mood disturbance was the primary measure in most studies. Among studies that reported group differences according to subscale, tension-anxiety and depression-dejection appeared to be the most sensitive in detecting differences between groups, showing an effect in three studies (Edbril & Rieker, 1989; Lerman et al., 1993; Magid & Golomb, 1989), whereas one report (Graydon, 1988) found differences only on tension-anxiety and another found them only on fatigue-inertia (Gritz, Wellisch, & Landsverk, 1988).

Several investigators found that distress lessened over time (Cassileth et al., 1989; Pozo et al., 1992; Waligora-Serafin et al., 1992). A number of studies confirmed the important influence of social factors on distress: higher distress was significantly correlated with employment-related problems (Edbril & Riecker, 1989; Magid & Golomb, 1989) and with problems related to social and family support (Cochran et al., 1987; Lichtman, Taylor, & Wood, 1987; Stam, Koopmans, & Mathieson, 1991).

Psychosocial Adjustment to Illness Scale. The PAIS (Derogatis, 1975b, 1986) provides a comprehensive assessment of adjustment to illness. It comes close to being a quality-of-life scale because of its multidimensional scope. However, we included it because it was developed to reflect adjustment in seven principal psychosocial areas. The PAIS is available in either an interview or self-report format, both of which contain 46 items. Respondents complete four-point scales with respect to the past 30 days. The scale yields seven subscales (see Table 1). It was originally validated on groups of individuals with a variety of acute and chronic illnesses, including lung and other cancers. Validation supported the internal consistency of the subscales as well as expected correlations with other scales, including the SCL-90-R. Scale scores also correlated well with clinicians' ratings.

A number of studies identified common correlates of negative PAIS scores, including internal attributions for the cause of cancer (Berckmann & Austin, 1993; Lowery, Jacobsen, & DuCette, 1993), recurrence of the disease (Cella, Mahon, & Donovan, 1990; Kornblith et al., 1992a), avoidant coping (Friedman et al., 1988b, 1990), and lack of social support (Friedman et al., 1988a; Gotcher, 1992; Northouse, 1988). Information about sex differences was inconsistent (Baider, Peretz, & Kaplan De-Nour, 1989; Carter, Carter, & Siliunas, 1993; Northouse & Swain, 1987). Two studies reported beneficial PAIS effects provided by an informational intervention (Durá & Ibañez, 1991) and adjuvant psychotherapy (Greer et al., 1992).

Psychometric Evaluation in Cancer Patients

Availability of psychometric information. Virtually every article reported data that are relevant to validity. Most reports provided a rationale for the choice of instruments, including discussions about reliability, validity, and use in comparable samples. Almost all of them used the instruments (in total or in selected subscales) as they had been developed; only one report (Pozo et al., 1992) extracted items from the parent scale (POMS) and created ad hoc subscales, including one subscale (friendliness) that does not correspond to any dimensions of the POMS. Although Pozo et al. presented information about the internal consistency of the subscales they created, the meaning of the subscales is questionable without additional analysis, especially for those with only two or three items. In a number of reports, predicted differences between groups and subscales support construct validation. However, only a few studies directly addressed validity and reliability issues, including a handful of additional articles that had scale validation as their specific objective.

Norms. Although most studies discussed findings in the context of standard norms or other studies with cancer patients, two developed norms specifically for the POMS. Cassileth et al. (1985) administered the POMS to 374 cancer patients and found that Total Mood Disturbance (TMD) was significantly less in the cancer patients (mean = 20.1) than in normative samples of psychotherapy patients (mean = 77.5) and college students (mean = 43.3). Cella et al. (1989) administered the POMS to 923 recently diagnosed cancer patients representing a variety of cancer sites and stages, and they reported both total and subscale scores. Cancer patients scored significantly lower than psychiatric outpatients and college students. However, their TMD mean of 37.0 differed from that obtained by Cassileth et al. (1985) in a similar sample.

Interrelationships among scales. Several studies addressed the interrelationships among scales. For example, Gritz et al. (1990) found that the POMS TMD and Depression-Dejection subscale and the CES-D were highly correlated (r = .91 and .87, respectively). In addition, the POMS subscales were relatively uncorrelated with the total POMS score except for the Depression-Dejection subscale. Jenkins, Linington, and Whittaker (1991) found that some PAIS subscales correlated well with subscales of the Hospital Anxiety and Depression Scale (HADS) (Zigmond & Snaith, 1983). Edgar, Rosberger, and Nowlis (1992) found that the CES-D was highly correlated with a number of other scales, including the Anxiety Scale of Lewis, Firisch, and Parsell (1979) and the Intrusion subscale from the Impact of Event (IOE) scale (Horowitz, Wilner, & Alvarez, 1979). Cassileth et al. (1989) found that the POMS and the BSI were strongly correlated at three time points (r = .71, .81, and .90). In Northouse and Swain's study (1987), the BSI and PAIS were strongly correlated (r = .68), although comparisons between patients and husbands revealed different response patterns in the two instruments. On the other hand, Baider, Peretz, and Kaplan De-Nour (1992) found that scores on the PAIS did not correlate well with those on the BSI and IOE scales for Holocaust survivors who had been diagnosed with cancer.

Greenwald (1987) compared the POMS to other scales often used in health assessment: the Sickness Impact Profile (SIP) (Bergner et al., 1976) and the McGill-Melzack Pain Inventory (Melzack, 1975). Greenwald based his study on 536 recently diagnosed cancer patients. Factor analyses indicated that each scale contributed distinct information about health; no single factor explained a preponderance of the variance, and the subscales of each scale generally loaded most strongly on individual factors corresponding to the parent scale. It should be noted that all the POMS subscales loaded highly on the "POMS factor" (loadings higher than .60), with the exception of the Vigor subscale, which loaded − .163 on the POMS factor but − .579 on the SIP factor.

Item aggregation. Several investigators who used multiple scales aggregated the item scores to form an overall score. Issues relating to this approach will be discussed later. Northouse (1988) used the BSI, the PAIS, and the Affects Balance Scale (Derogatis, 1975c). Raw scores were converted to standard scores and summed to form an overall adjustment score. Stam, Koopmans, and Mathieson (1991) administered the CES-D, the POMS short form (Shacham, 1983), and the STAI and created composite distress scores by summing the scores. A factor analysis indicated that a single factor explained .91 of the variance in scores. Bloom et al. (1987) included a number of self-report instruments (including the BSI and four other scales), observer-rated scales, and content analysis scales. All the scores were subjected to a principal components analysis, which yielded seven components, three derived from the self-report instruments: psychopathology, negative attitude, and somatic distress. These components were then used as the dependent variables in multivariate analyses of variance. Lichtman, Taylor, and Wood (1987) used 10 different self-report measures, including the POMS, and found that one principal factor accounted for 76 percent of the variance.

Development of POMS short forms. Three reports examined the POMS in an effort to reduce its length, examine its factor structure, or both. Interestingly, each research team took a different approach, and the resultant shortened scales were largely nonoverlapping. Shacham (1983) used a sample of 83 cancer patients to develop a shortened version of the POMS. Items that had low coefficient alphas were dropped; the result was a 37-item scale, each subscale of which correlated .95 or better with the original POMS. Although we could not identify any studies that examined the factor structure of the brief scale, such work is in progress (personal communication, Barbara Curbow, PhD, The Johns Hopkins University, February 1994). Stam, Koopmans, and Mathieson (1991) used the short form in an independent sample; however, they did not report information about the scale but instead used it as part of an overall distress factor, as was discussed earlier.

Cella et al. (1987) developed a measure of TMD based on 11 items from the original POMS and administered it to 619 patients with cancers other than lung cancer. A principal components factor analysis specifying one factor was conducted, and 11 items with high loadings on this factor were retained as a short form, which manifested high internal consistency. The items in the short form reflected five of the six original POMS subscales, thus supporting its multidimensionality. A replication sample of 295 lung cancer patients confirmed the comparability of findings and the correlation between the long and short forms of the POMS and the high internal consistency of the short form. Comparisons across cancer sites supported the comparability of findings between the short and long POMS. No studies using Cella et al.'s form were identified.

Guadagnoli and Mor (1989) used a different approach. Their aims were (1) to examine whether two underlying dimensions—positive and negative affect—rather than the six subscales proposed could adequately describe the scale and (2) to develop a shortened version of the scale. They conducted a factor analysis using the POMS scores of two samples: 438 newly diagnosed lung, breast, and colorectal patients and 225 patients receiving chemotherapy. A principal components analysis on half the patients in the first sample revealed two major components corresponding to positive and negative affect. This solution was replicated in other patient samples. Guadagnoli and Mor used the item loadings on the two factors (those that loaded highly on one factor and low on the other) as well as eliminating items with somatic content to identify the best set of items for an abbreviated scale; this process yielded 14 items (7 positive and 7 negative). Although the investigators concluded that their two-factor solution was supported, they also reported that the two subscales were significantly negatively correlated (− .34) in one patient sample but not in the other. This finding indicates the need for additional testing in other patient samples. However, we did not identify any studies that have used the Guadagnoli and Mor's short form of the POMS.

When individual items are compared across the three shortened scales, only one, "blue," is found in all three questionnaires! Seven of Cella et al.'s 11 items and 5 of Guadagnoli and Mor's 14 items overlap with the items included by Shacham. Only one item is the same in Cella et al.'s and Guadagnoli and Mor's short forms. These findings should not be viewed as completely contradictory (although more overlap among scales might have been expected). Instead, the two short forms reflect the different analytic purposes of the investigators; they also illustrate how a researcher must be careful to select not just a "short POMS" but, rather, an instrument that is congruent with the conceptual underpinnings of the specific study.

Development of new scales. Several investigators used scales cited in this review to validate new scales. Noyes et al. (1990) used the BDI for a new scale of cancer-related distress, and Bisno and Richardson (1987) used it for scales of pleasant and unpleasant events. Bruera et al. (1989) used the SCL-90-R to validate a scale of asthenia (or fatigue). Sutherland, Lockwood, and Cunningham (1989) used the POMS and the SCL-90-R to validate a new POMS Linear Analogue Scale (LASA), which included one linear analogue scale corresponding to each POMS subscale. Forty-two patients with mixed cancers completed the three instruments before and after participating in a coping skills intervention. Their study found a high correlation between the POMS and the SCL-90-R (79 percent of the variance in SCL-90-R scores could be explained by the six POMS subscale scores). Furthermore, Sutherland et al. found that the POMS LASA was highly correlated with both of the other scales and was sensitive to changes before and after the intervention. They concluded that the POMS dimensions may address more stable aspects of affect than transient mood, that the somatic content of the POMS items does not detract from their sensitivity with cancer patients, and that brief scales such as the POMS LASA may be as effective as more intensive assessment strategies.

Predictive validity. Two teams used POMS scores as an indicator of "high distress" and attempted to predict POMS scores on the basis of other factors. When Zabora et al. (1990) used the BSI and the Inventory of Current Concerns (ICC) (Weisman & Worden, 1976) to identify patients with problems on the POMS, the PAIS, or both 9 to 12 months later, they found that the BSI and the ICC were highly correlated and recommended the BSI as a screening instrument because of its relative simplicity. The BSI correctly identified future distress in 84 percent of patients. Their report did not describe how "negative results" were defined for the POMS or the PAIS; these definitions are important, however, because cutoff points that correspond to clinical distress are not included in the instruments. In addition, the POMS and the PAIS were not administered at baseline; given the high intercorrelations found by other investigators among all these instruments, it is important to determine whether the BSI exhibited test-retest reliability over time because of its relationship with the POMS, the PAIS, or both or because it indicated new cases of distress. Pruitt et al. (1991), who also used the ICC as a predictor for POMS scores three and six months after baseline, raised this possibility. The ICC was not successful in predicting distress in their sample, and POMS scores remained relatively stable over the two time points.

Multimethod approaches. Although little research has focused on relationships between scale scores and other sources of data, there are several interesting exceptions. Bloom et al. (1990) assessed the correlation between the POMS Vigor and Fatigue subscales and the energy expended to perform leisure and work activities. The energy requirements of various activities had already been established, and 85 survivors of Hodgkin's disease were asked to report on their activity patterns and to complete the POMS scales. Bloom et al. found that the POMS scores correlated well with activity patterns and specifically with the energy expended for discretionary leisure activities but not for work activities. This finding provides support for the construct validation of the POMS, although the self-report and retrospective nature of both assessments should be noted. Heinrich and Schag (1987) used prospective patient diaries to document activity levels, which was useful in interpreting other findings.

Finally, Fawzy et al. (1990a, 1990b) presented an exciting advance in assessment methods. Sixty-six newly diagnosed patients with malignant melanoma were randomly assigned to a short-term psychiatric group intervention or to a control condition. They were assessed at baseline, six weeks later at the end of the intervention, and six months after that. Several measures were used: the POMS to measure affect; a coping inventory; and assessments of immunological functioning. In brief, the intervention led to positive mood changes as well as beneficial changes in immune functioning; evidence suggested that these changes were mediated by coping methods. Furthermore, the POMS correlated with immune functioning. Fawzy et al. stressed that additional research was needed to replicate, clarify, and extend their findings. This approach constitutes an interesting challenge for psychosocial oncology research.

DISCUSSION

This review has several limitations. Not all psychological functioning scales of interest were cited in research published in the *Journal of Psychosocial Oncology*. In particular, one scale that has been used extensively with European cancer patients, the HADS, did not appear often enough to list. In addition, the time frame excluded earlier relevant articles. We also are aware that the studies we selected do not represent all the relevant articles.

This article demonstrates that the seven instruments reviewed have been used in a variety of patient samples and have provided useful information. However, a large amount of inconsistency exists in study findings and psychometric evaluations. Although some inconsistencies can be attributed to variation in study samples and designs, some are likely to be the result of measurement error as well. Several specific areas of concern are discussed below.

Lack of psychometric information. As we discussed earlier, only a few researchers reported validation information in cancer patient samples. Although most investigators have not indicated examining the psychometric properties of the scales we urge them to do so; psychometric information can be obtained even within a study that is not explicitly directed toward this purpose. For example, given sufficient numbers of cases, a confirmatory factor analysis can be undertaken to examine the replicability of the factor structure of a scale. The substantial variation in current results casts considerable doubt about the replicability of the subscales of the various instruments. Confirmatory factor analyses conducted for various scales have helped to clarify the stability of their structure and the need for population-specific adaptations. For example, such analyses have supported the validity of the BSI in Chinese samples (Chan, 1991), identified the need to modify the CES-D to make it appropriate for samples of American Indians (Beals et al., 1991) and Hispanics (Guarnaccia, Angel, & Worobey, 1989), and pointed out concerns about using the SCL-90-R for patients with posttraumatic stress disorder (Schwarzwald, Weisenberg, & Solomon, 1991) and the BSI with psychiatric patients (Boulet & Boss, 1991). Scale validation is a continuous process and is especially important for scales used in groups such as cancer patients, which differ from the original validation samples.

Norms. The availability of normative information against which to compare study results provides a strong incentive for using a particular scale. For example, if norms for psychiatric populations are available, one can judge whether a given cancer patient (or group of patients) is relatively more distressed than are individuals who need psychiatric care. However, answering this question may not be the aim of the study. The "threshold" for "need for psychological or psychiatric consultation" may be different for cancer patients than for other groups. The use of inappropriate normative information may confer conclusions and interpretations that are not congruent with clinical reality for cancer patients. Thus, investigators should critically weigh the interpretation of specific norms relative to the study objectives. If their aim is to identify cancer patients who are at particular risk, norms based on psychiatric samples may be useless. As we discussed earlier, several researchers have established cancer patient norms for the POMS (Cassileth et al., 1985; Cella et al., 1989), although the lack of consistency between these norms points out the difficulty of developing and interpreting such data.

Content validity. The seven scales, all of which were initially reported at least a decade ago, were developed primarily in psychiatric or student populations, although the PAIS included cancer patients early in the validation process. This process raises a question about the content validity of these scales: To what degree are items on the scales applicable to cancer patients? The issue of the somatic content of many scale items is often raised: for example, the BSI includes questions about symptoms such as weight loss and sleeping difficulties. Although these symptoms may reflect depression in physically healthy populations, they may be confounded by cancer and its treatment. Researchers should carefully consider whether a scale is appropriate for their population of cancer patients.

A related concern regarding content validity that has been raised less often is the extent to which the scales reflect the aspects of psychological functioning that are important to cancer patients. After their development, the scales have been used "as is" with other specialized populations. As such, their use with cancer patients omits the critical first step in the development of an instrument–the item-generation phase, which should be based on the important dimensions identified by members of the target population and by other individuals with relevant expertise. Some aspects of psychological distress may be distinct in cancer and perhaps other life-threatening diseases: for example, spiritual concerns (see Jenkins and Pargament, this volume). Or perhaps symptoms such as depression and anxiety may assume different weights in cancer patients; thus a summated scale does not reflect the degree of dysfunction that is actually experienced. Distinct concerns of subgroups, such as patients from different ethnic and cultural backgrounds, also need to be considered in judging the appropriateness of a scale and developing or adapting the scale as necessary. Future research should evaluate these concerns about content validity. Using systematic semistructured interviews with cancer patients, families, and care providers is one way to ensure that questionnaire items are derived from the perspectives of the target populations rather than from those of the researcher. Scales developed for cancer patients, such as Noyes et al.'s Illness Distress Scale (1990),

McCorkle and Young's Symptom Distress Scale (1978), and the Rotterdam Symptom Checklist (de Haes, van Knippenberg, & Neijt, 1990) may provide useful information in this regard.

Item aggregation. The most common use of factor analysis in the studies reviewed here was to aggregate the multiple scales and subscales originally included into a single, presumably more interpretable measure, which was then subjected to analysis. Clearly, considerable overlap exists across scales, and a number of studies found a single "distress" factor was common across the data from their many measures. High levels of variance on the resultant distress scores can be explained by the factor. Given the multiple items that comprise them, aggregated scores also tend to be more stable than are scores based on fewer items. These features add to the psychometric attractiveness of this approach.

However, the attractive statistical aspects of this strategy need to be balanced against its conceptual contributions. Combining all study information into a single score means that a large amount of potentially valuable information is lost. A number of the studies reviewed here found useful differences among the different questionnaires and subscales. With only a single factor, psychosocial oncology researchers are left with gross ratings of overall distress rather than being able to pinpoint specific areas of concern. This may hinder rather than facilitate study interpretation. The issue of how many factors are required to describe a construct adequately is not limited to psychosocial oncology; it is an area of spirited debate among mood and personality theorists (Goldberg, 1993; McConville & Cooper, 1992). Additional research and theory building is needed to clarify these concerns.

Item reduction. Few researchers examined their scales to identify the best questions or scales, reduce redundancy, and enable future researchers to test a new scale composed of a subset of the best items. Without this information, researchers remain in the position of having to administer all of the same scales even though doing so is inefficient. Given comparable information obtained, the shorter scale is preferred, particularly because of cancer patients' physical limitations and the resultant burden of providing data. However, even when researchers have developed short forms such as the brief POMS (Cella et al., 1987; Guadagnoli & Mor, 1989; Shacham,

1983; Sutherland, Lockwood, & Cunningham, 1989), these scales apparently are not widely used. Similarly, it is unclear why investigators would choose to use the SCL-90-R when the BSI, a much briefer instrument that yields parallel information, is available.

Study samples. The overwhelming number of studies reviewed here used breast cancer patients. This homogeneity allows some control for disease and treatment-related variables and reflects psychosocial oncology researchers' increased sophistication about the importance of medical aspects of cancer. At the time, however, the lack of diverse patient populations limits the generalizability of findings to other cancers. One obvious limitation is the lack of knowledge about psychological functioning in men and, by implication, about sex differences. Why breast cancer is studied so often is easy to understand, given its high prevalence and intense psychosocial impact. It is also true that much remains to be learned about breast cancer patients' psychological well-being and how to promote it. However, the time has come for researchers to extend their scope, especially to other cancers with a high prevalence, such as lung, prostate, and colorectal cancers.

Interpretation. Investigators are urged to continue exploring the interpretation of scale scores. Such information is vitally important not only to research but also to clinical care. Several scales have developed cutoff points, which identify patients who are likely to be clinically distressed or require full clinical evaluation. This kind of information is extremely important to distinguish between statistically and clinically significant information and to provide a basis for using the scales in the care of individual patients. However, little attention has focused on developing a correspondence between scale scores and clinical factors or exploring whether cutoffs developed for other populations are meaningful for cancer patients. For example, of the patients judged to be clinically distressed on the BSI, how many were found to be depressed in clinical practice? Spiegel and Sands (1988) and Carpenter, Morrow, and Schmale (1989) reported initial results comparing self-report scales to clinical interview data, which represent a useful beginning to addressing the issue. In addition, the use of scales in intervention studies will help determine their clinical usefulness. The vast majority of the studies in Table 2 are descriptive.

Use of self-report data. Finally, investigators need to consider the validity of assessing psychological distress through self-reports. Shedler, Mayman, and Manis (1993) have questioned whether self-reports are sensitive enough to uncover real problems experienced by patients and have cited numerous examples of self-reports that significantly underreport clinical problems. According to Shedler and colleagues, psychological denial contributes a strong and pervasive bias in self-reports of psychological functioning. Cancer patients may experience additional pressure to present themselves positively because they may not want to be viewed as complainers, or "bad patients." In fact, some research has demonstrated the influence of social desirability on cancer patients' self-reports of quality of life (Hürny et al., 1987), and several articles reviewed here have mentioned the possibility that social desirability, denial, or both may have affected their results (Carpenter, Morrow, & Schmale, 1989; Guadagnoli & Mor, 1989). Concern about the validity of self-reports is certainly not specific to psychosocial oncology. Additional approaches to self-reports, such as self-monitoring and role playing, may be useful. In addition, all psychosocial researchers need to consider triangulation of assessment measures—that is, obtain complementary information from different sources such as observer ratings, actual behaviors, and psychophysiological measures (Turpin, 1989) to obtain a full and accurate picture of patient functioning. Fawzy et al.'s work (1990a, 1990b) represents an example of this approach. Although such research can be costly and time consuming, the same can be said about research that uses self-report instruments. The meaningfulness and interpretability of an assessment tool ultimately determine its cost-benefit ratio.

The field of psychosocial oncology, and outcome assessment in particular, has come a long way. A decade ago, this review would not have been possible. The studies reviewed here used some of the best tools available when the research was conducted. However, many challenges remain in the pursuit of valid and reliable assessments of psychological functioning in cancer patients. Critical attention to issues such as those raised in this article will lead to considerable progress toward this goal over the next decade as "second-generation" instruments are developed and tested.

REFERENCES

American Cancer Society. (1984). Proceedings of the Working Conference on Methodology in Behavioral and Psychosocial Cancer Research. *Cancer, 53*(Suppl.), 2217-2284.

Anastasi, A. (1988). *Psychological testing* (6th ed.). New York: Macmillan.

Baider, L., & Kaplan De-Nour, A. (1986). The meaning of disease: An exploratory study of Moslem Arab women after a mastectomy. *Journal of Psychosocial Oncology, 4*(4), 1-15.

Baider, L., Peretz, T., & Kaplan De-Nour, A. (1989). Gender and adjustment to chronic disease: A study of couples with colon cancer. *General Hospital Psychiatry 11(1)*, 1-8.

Baider, L., Peretz, T., & Kaplan De-Nour, A. (1992). Effect of the Holocaust on coping with cancer. *Social Science & Medicine, 34*(1), 11-15.

Beals, J., Manson, S. M., Keane, E. M., & Dick, R. W. (1991). Factorial structure of the Center for Epidemiological Studies–Depression Scale among American Indian college students. *Psychological Assessment, 3*, 623-627.

Bech, P. (1992). Symptoms and assessment of depression. In E. S. Paykel (Ed.), *Handbook of affective disorders* (pp. 3-14). New York: Guilford Press.

Beck, A. T., & Beamesderfer, A. (1974). Assessment of depression: The Depression Inventory. In P. Pichot (Ed.), *Psychological measurements in psychopharmacology* (pp. 151-169). Basel, Switzerland: S. Karger.

Beck, A. T., Ward, C. H., Mendelson, M., Mock, J., & Erbaugh, J. (1961). An inventory for measuring depression. *Archives of General Psychiatry, 4*, 561-571.

Berckman, K. L., & Austin, J. K. (1993). Causal attribution, perceived control, and adjustment in patients with lung cancer. *Oncology Nursing Forum, 20*, 23-30.

Bergner, M., Bobbitt, R. A., Pollard, W. E., Martin, D. P., & Gilson, B. S. (1976). Sickness Impact Profile: Validation of a health status measure. *Medical Care, 14*(1), 57-67.

Bisno, B., & Richardson, J. L. (1987). The relationship between depression and reinforcing events in cancer patients. *Journal of Psychosocial Oncology, 5*(2), 63-71.

Bloom, J. R., Cook, M., Fotopoulis, S., Flamer, D., Gates, C., Holland, J. C., Meunze, L. R., Murawski, B., Penman, D., & Ross, R. D. (1987). Psychological response to mastectomy. *Cancer, 59*, 189-196.

Bloom, J. R., Hoppe, R. T., Fobair, P., Cox, R. S., Varghese, A., & Spiegel, D. (1988). Effects of treatment on the work experiences of long-term survivors of Hodgkin's disease. *Journal of Psychosocial Oncology, 6*(3/4), 65-80.

Bloom, J. R., Gorsky, R. D., Fobair, P., Hoppe, R., Cox, R. S., Varghese, A., & Spiegel, D. (1990). Physical performance at work and at leisure: Validation of a measure of biological energy in survivors of Hodgkin's disease. *Journal of Psychosocial Oncology, 8*(1), 49-63.

Boulet, J., & Boss, M. W. (1991). Reliability and validity of the Brief Symptom Inventory. *Psychological Assessment, 3*, 433-437.

Bruera, E., Brenneis, C., Michaud, M., Rafter, J., Magnan, A., Tennant, A., Hanson, J., & Macdonald, R. N. (1989). Association between asthenia and nutritional status, lean body mass, anemia, psychological status, and tumor mass in patients with advanced breast cancer. *Journal of Pain & Symptom Management, 4*(2), 59-63.

Carpenter, P. J., Morrow, G. R., & Schmale, A. H. (1989). The psychosocial status of cancer patients after cessation of treatment. *Journal of Psychosocial Oncology, 7*(1/2), 95-103.

Carter, R. E., Carter, C. A., & Siliunas, M. (1993). Marital adaptation and interaction of couples after a mastectomy. *Journal of Psychosocial Oncology, 11*(2), 69-82.

Cassileth, B. R., Lusk, E. J., Brown, L. L., & Cross, P. A. (1985). Psychosocial status of cancer patients and next of kin: Normative data from the Profile of Mood States. *Journal of Psychosocial Oncology, 3*(3), 99-105.

Cassileth, B. R., Lusk, E. J., Walsh, W. P., Doyle, B., & Maier, M. (1989). The satisfaction and psychosocial status of patients during treatment for cancer. *Journal of Psychosocial Oncology, 7*(4), 47-57.

Cella, D. F., & Tulsky, D. S. (1990). Measuring quality of life today: Methodological aspects. *Oncology, 4*(5), 29-38.

Cella, D. F., Mahon, S. M., & Donovan, M. I. (1990). Cancer recurrence as a traumatic event. *Behavioral Medicine, 16*, 15-22.

Cella, D. F., Jacobsen, P. B., Orav, E. J., Holland, J. C., Silberfarb, P. M., & Rafla, S. (1987). A brief POMS measure of distress for cancer patients. *Journal of Chronic Diseases, 40*, 939-942.

Cella, D. F., Tross, S., Orav, E. J., Holland, J. C., Silberfarb, P. M., & Rafla, S. (1989). Mood states of patients after the diagnosis of cancer. *Journal of Psychosocial Oncology, 7*(1/2), 45-54.

Challis, G. B., & Stam, H. J. (1992). A longitudinal study of the development of anticipatory nausea and vomiting in cancer chemotherapy patients: The role of absorption and autonomic perception. *Health Psychology, 11*, 181-189.

Chan, D. F. (1991). The Beck Depression Inventory: What difference does the Chinese version make? *Psychological Assessment, 3*, 616-622.

Cochran, S. D., Hacker, N. F., Wellisch, D. K., & Berek, J. S. (1987). Sexual function after treatment for endometrial cancer. *Journal of Psychosocial Oncology, 5*(2), 47-61.

Cull, A. M. (1992). The assessment of sexual function in cancer patients. *European Journal of Cancer, 28A*, 1680-1686.

Curbow, B., & Somerfield, M. (1991). Use of the Rosenberg Self-Esteem Scale with adult cancer patients. *Journal of Psychosocial Oncology, 9*(2), 113-131.

deHaes, J. C. J. M., van Knippenberg, F. C. E., & Neijt, J. P. (1990). Measuring psychological and physical distress in cancer patients: Structure and application of the Rotterdam Symptom Checklist. *British Journal of Cancer, 62*, 1034-1038.

Derogatis, L. R. (1975a). *Brief Symptom Inventory.* Baltimore, MD: Clinical Psychometric Research.

Derogatis, L. R. (1975b). *Psychosocial Adjustment to Illness Scale.* Baltimore, MD: Clinical Psychometric Research.

Derogatis, L. R. (1975c). *Affects Balance Scale.* Baltimore, MD: Clinical Psychometric Research.

Derogatis, L. R. (1977). *SCL-90-R: Administration, scoring, and procedures manual-I.* Baltimore, MD: Clinical Psychometric Research.

Derogatis, L. R. (1986). The Psychosocial Adjustment to Illness Scale (PAIS). *Journal of Psychosomatic Research, 30*(1), 77-91.

Derogatis, L. R., & Melisaratos, N. (1983). The Brief Symptom Inventory: An introductory report. *Psychological Medicine, 13*, 595-605.

Derogatis, L. R., & Wise, T. N. (Eds.). (1989). *Anxiety and depressive disorders in the medical patient.* Washington, DC: American Psychiatric Press.

DeVellis, R. F. (1991). *Scale development, theory, and applications.* Newbury Park, CA: Sage Publications.

Durà, E., & Ibañez, E. (1991). The psychosocial effects of an information program involving Spanish breast cancer patients. *Journal of Psychosocial Oncology, 9*(2), 45-65.

Edbril, S. D., & Rieker, P. P. (1989). The impact of testicular cancer on the work lives of survivors. *Journal of Psychosocial Oncology, 7*(3), 17-29.

Edgar, L., Rosberger, Z., & Nowlis, D. (1992). Coping with cancer during the first year after diagnosis. *Cancer, 69*, 817-828.

Fawzy, F. I., Cousins, N., Fawzy, N. W., Kemeny, M. E., Elashoff, R., & Morton, C. (1990a). A structured psychiatric intervention for cancer patients: I. Changes over time in methods of coping and affective disturbance. *Archives of General Psychiatry, 47*, 720-725.

Fawzy, F. I., Kemeny, M. E., Fawzy, N. W., Elashoff, R., Morton, D., Cousins, N., & Fahey, J. L. (1990b). A structured psychiatric intervention for cancer patients: II. Changes over time in immunological measures. *Archives of General Psychiatry, 47*, 729-735.

Fobair, P., Hoppe, R. T., & Bloom, J. R. (1986). Psychosocial problems among survivors of Hodgkin's disease. *Journal of Clinical Oncology, 4*, 805-814.

Friedman, L. C., Baer, P. E., Lewy, A., Lane, M., & Smith, F. E. (1988a). Predictors of psychosocial adjustment to breast cancer. *Journal of Psychosocial Oncology, 6*(1/2), 75-94.

Friedman, L. C., Baer, P. E., Nelson, D. V., Lane, M., Smith, F. E., & Dworkin, R. J. (1988b). Women with breast cancer: Perception of family functioning and adjustment to illness. *Psychosomatic Medicine, 50*, 529-540.

Friedman, L. C., Nelson, D. V., Baer, P. E., Lane, M., & Smith, F. E. (1990). Adjustment to breast cancer: A replication study. *Journal of Psychosocial Oncology, 8*(4), 27-40.

Gilbar, O. (1989). Who refuses chemotherapy? A profile. *Psychological Reports, 64*, 1291-1297.

Gilbar, O. (1991). The quality of life of cancer patients who refuse chemotherapy. *Social Science & Medicine, 32*, 1337-1340.

Gilbar, O., & Florian, V. (1991). Do women with inoperable breast cancer have a psychological profile? *Omega Journal of Death & Dying, 23*, 217-226.

Gilbar, O., & Kaplan De-Nour, A. (1989). Adjustment to illness and dropout of chemotherapy. *Journal of Psychosomatic Research, 33*(1), 1-5.

Goldberg, L. R. (1993). The structure of phenotypic personality traits. *American Psychologist, 48*(1), 26-34.

Goldstein, A., & Herson, M. (Eds.). (1990). *Handbook of psychological assessment* (2nd ed.). New York: Pergamon Press.

Gotcher, J. M. (1992). Interpersonal communication and psychosocial adjustment. *Journal of Psychosocial Oncology, 10*, 21-39.

Gottschalk, L. A. (1984). Measurement of mood and affect in cancer patients. *Cancer, 53*, 2236-2242.

Graydon, J. E. (1988). Factors that predict patients' functioning following treatment for cancer. *International Journal of Nursing Studies, 25*, 117-124.

Greenwald, H. P. (1987). The specificity of quality-of-life measures among the seriously ill. *Medical Care, 25*, 642-651.

Greer, S., Moorey, S., Baruch, J. D. R., Watson, M., Robertson, B. M., Mason, A., Rowden, L., Law, M. E., & Bliss, J. M. (1992). Adjuvant psychological therapy for patients with cancer: A prospective randomised trial. *British Medical Journal, 304*, 675-680.

Gritz, E. R., Wellisch, D. K., & Landsverk, J. A. (1988). Psychosocial sequelae in long-term survivors of testicular cancer. *Journal of Psychosocial Oncology, 6*(3/4), 41-63.

Gritz, E. R., Wellisch, D. K., Siau, J., & Wang, H. J. (1990). Long-term effects of testicular cancer on marital relationships. *Psychosomatics, 31*, 301-312.

Guadagnoli, E., & Mor, V. (1989). Profile of Mood States (POMS). *Psychological Assessment, 1*, 150-154.

Guarnaccia, P. J., Angel, R., & Worobey, J. L. (1989). The factor structure of the CES-D in the Hispanic Health and Nutrition Examination Survey: The influences of ethnicity, gender and language. *Social Science & Medicine, 29*, 85-94.

Hannum, J. W., Geiss-Davis, J., Harding, K., & Hatfield, A. K. (1991). Effects of individual and marital variables on coping with cancer. *Journal of Psychosocial Oncology, 9*(2), 1-20.

Haut, M. W., Beckwith, B. E., Laurie, J. A., & Klatt, N. (1991). Postchemotherapy nausea and vomiting in cancer patients receiving outpatient chemotherapy. *Journal of Psychosocial Oncology, 9*(1), 117-130.

Heim, H. M., & Oei, T. P. S. (1993). Comparison of prostate cancer patients with and without pain. *Pain, 53*, 159-162.

Heinrich, R. L., & Schag, C. C. (1987). The psychosocial impact of cancer: Cancer patients and healthy controls. *Journal of Psychosocial Oncology, 5*(2), 75-91.

Hopwood, P. (1993). The assessment of body image in cancer patients. *European Journal of Cancer, 29A*, 276-281.

Horowitz, M., Wilner, N., & Alvarez, W. (1979). Impact of Event Scale: A measure of subjective stress. *Psychosomatic Medicine, 41*, 209-218.

Hürny, C., Piasetsky, E., Bagin, R., & Holland, J. (1987). High social desirability in patients being treated for advanced colorectal cancer: Eventual impact on the assessment of quality of life. *Journal of Psychosocial Oncology, 5*(1), 19-29.

Hursti, T., Fredrikson, M., Börjeson, S., Fürst, C. J., Peterson, C., & Steineck, G. (1992). Association between personality characteristics and the prevalence and extinction of conditioned nausea after chemotherapy. *Journal of Psychosocial Oncology, 10*(2), 59-77.

Irwin, P. H., Kramer, S., Diamond, N. H., Malone, D., & Zivin, G. (1986). Sex differences in psychological distress during definitive radiation therapy for cancer. *Journal of Psychosocial Oncology, 4*(3), 63-73.

Irwin, P. H., & Kramer, S. (1988). Social support and cancer: Sustained emotional support and successful adaptation. *Journal of Psychosocial Oncology, 6*(1/2), 63-73.

Jenkins, P. L., Linington, A., & Whittaker, J. A. (1991). A retrospective study of psychosocial morbidity in bone marrow transplant recipients. *Psychosomatics, 32(1)*, 65-71.

Johnstone, B. G. M., Silberfield, M., Chapman, J., Phoenix, C., Sturgeon, J. F. G., Till, J. E., & Sutcliffe, S. B. (1991). Heterogeneity in responses to cancer. Part I: Psychiatric Symptoms. *Canadian Journal of Psychiatry, 36*, 85-90.

Kornblith, A. B., Anderson, J., Cella, D. F., Tross, S., Zuckerman, E., Cherin, E., Henderson, E., Canellos, G. P., Kosty, M. P., Cooper, M. R., Weiss, R. B., Gottlieb, A., & Holland, J. C. (1992a). Comparison of psychosocial adaptation and sexual function of survivors of advanced Hodgkin disease treated by MOPP, ABVD, or MOPP alternating with ABVD. *Cancer, 70*, 2508-2516.

Kornblith, A. B., Anderson, J., Cella, D. F., Tross, S., Zuckerman, E., Cherin, E., Henderson, E., Canellos, G. P., Kosty, M. P., Cooper, M. R., Weiss, R. B., Gottlieb, A., & Holland, J. C. (1992b). Hodgkin disease survivors at increased risk for problems in psychosocial adaptation. *Cancer, 70*, 2214-2224.

Kukull, W. A., McCorkle, R., & Driever, M. (1986). Symptom distress, psychosocial variables, and survival from lung cancer. *Journal of Psychosocial Oncology, 4*(1/2), 91-104.

Leinster, S. J., Ashcroft, J. J., Slade, P. D., & Dewey, M. E. (1989). Mastectomy versus conservative surgery: Psychosocial effects of the patient's choice of treatment. *Journal of Psychosocial Oncology, 7*(1/2), 179-192.

Lerman, C., Daly, M., Walsh, W. P., Resch, N., Seay, J., Barsevick, A., Birenbaum, L., Heggan, T., & Martin, G. (1993). Communication between patients with breast cancer and health care providers. *Cancer, 72*, 2612-2620.

Lewis, F. M., Firisch, S. C., & Parsell, S. (1979). Clinical tool development for adult chemotherapy patients: Process and content. *Cancer Nursing, 2*, 99-108.

Lichtman, R. R., Taylor, S. E., & Wood, J. V. (1987). Social support and marital adjustment after breast cancer. *Journal of Psychosocial Oncology, 5*(3), 47-74.

Locke, H. J., & Wallace, K. M. (1959). Short marital adjustment and prediction tests: Their reliability and validity. *Marriage & Family Living, 21*, 251-255.

Lowery, B. M., Jacobsen, B. S., & DuCette, J. (1993). Causal attribution, control, and adjustment to breast cancer. *Journal of Psychosocial Oncology, 10*(4), 37-53.

Magid, D. M., & Golomb, H. (1989). Effect of employment on coping with chronic illness among patients with hairy cell leukemia. *Journal of Psychosocial Oncology, 7*(1/2), 1-17.

McConville, C., & Cooper, C. (1992). The structure of moods. *Personality & Individual Differences, 13*, 909-919.

McCorkle, R., & Young, K. (1978). Development of a symptom distress scale. *Cancer Nursing, 1*, 373-378.

McNair, D. M., Lorr, M., & Droppleman, L. F. (1971). *EDITS manual for the Profile of Mood States.* San Diego, CA: Education and Industrial Testing Service.

Melzack, R. (1975). The McGill Pain Questionnaire: Major properties and scoring methods. *Pain, 1*, 227-229.

Morrow, G. R. (1992). Behavioural factors influencing the development and expression of chemotherapy induced side effects. *British Journal of Cancer, 66*(Suppl.), S54-S61.

Nayfield, S. G., Hailey, B. J., & McCabe, M. (1990, July 16-17). *Report of the Workshop on Quality of Life Research in Cancer Clinical Trials,* co-sponsored by the National Cancer Institute and the Office of Medical Applications of Research, National Institutes of Health, Bethesda, MD.

Northouse, L. L. (1988). Social support in patients' and husbands' adjustment to breast cancer. *Nursing Research, 37*, 91-95.

Northouse, L. L., & Swain, M. A. (1987). Adjustment of patients and their husbands to the initial impact of breast cancer. *Nursing Research, 36*, 221-225.

Noyes, R., Kathol, R. G., Debelius-Enemark, P., Williams, J., Mutgi, A., Suelzer, M. T., & Clamon, G. H. (1990). Distress associated with cancer as measured by the Illness Distress Scale. *Psychosomatics, 31*, 321-330.

Nunnally, J. C., & Bernstein, I. H. (1994). *Psychometric theory.* New York: McGraw-Hill.

Oberst, M. T., & Scott, D. W. (1988). Postdischarge distress in surgically treated cancer patients and their spouses. *Research in Nursing & Health, 11*, 223-233.

Pozo, C., Carver, C. S., Noriega, V., Harris, S. D., Robinson, D. S., Ketcham, A. S., Legaspi, A., Moffat, F. L., & Clark, K. C. (1992). Effects of mastectomy versus lumpectomy on emotional adjustment to breast cancer: A prospective study of the first year postsurgery. *Journal of Clinical Oncology, 10*, 1292-1298.

Pruitt, B. T., Waligora-Serafin, B., McMahon, T., & Davenport, J. (1991). Prediction of distress in the first six months after a cancer diagnosis. *Journal of Psychosocial Oncology, 9*(4), 91-102.

Quinn, M. E., Fontana, A. F., & Reznikoff, M. (1986). Psychological distress in reaction to lung cancer as a function of spousal support and coping strategy. *Journal of Psychosocial Oncology, 4*(4), 79-90.

Rabkin, J. G., & Klein, D. F. (1987). The clinical measurement of depressive disorders. In A. J. Marsella, R. M. A. Hirschfeld, & M. M. Katz (Eds.), *The measurement of depression* (pp. 30-79). New York: Guilford Press.

Roberts, C. S., Baile, W. F., Jr., Elkins, N. W., & Cox, C. E. (1990). Effects of interview context on the assessment of mood in breast cancer patients: A replication study. *Journal of Psychosocial Oncology, 8*(1), 33-47.

Roberts, C. S., Rossetti, K., Cone, D., & Cavanagh, D. (1992). Psychosocial impact of gynecologic cancer: A descriptive study. *Journal of Psychosocial Oncology, 10*(1), 99-109.

Schwarzwald, J., Weisenberg, M., & Solomon, Z. (1991). Factor invariance of SCL-90-R: The case of combat stress reaction. *Psychological Assessment, 3*, 385-390.

Shacham, S. (1983). A shortened version of the Profile of Mood States. *Journal of Personality Assessment, 47*, 305-306.

Shedler, J., Mayman, M., & Manis, M. (1993). The *illusion* of mental health. *American Psychologist, 48*, 1117-1131.

Silverman-Dresner, T. (1989-90). Self-help groups for women who have had breast cancer. *Imagination, Cognition, & Personality, 9*, 237-243.

Silverman-Dresner, T., & Restaino-Baumann, L. (1989-90). Problems associated with mastectomy. *Imagination, Cognition & Personality, 9*, 157-176.

Silverman-Dresner, T., & Restaino-Baumann, L. (1990-91). Comparison of symptom profiles between postmastectomy patients and normally healthy middle-aged women. *Imagination, Cognition, & Personality, 10*, 195-200.

Sneed, N.V., Edlund, B., & Dias, J. K. (1992). Adjustment of gynecological and breast cancer patients to the cancer diagnosis: Comparisons with males and females having other cancer sites. *Health Care for Women International, 13*, 11-22.

Spiegel, D., & Sands, S. H. (1988). Pain management in the cancer patient. *Journal of Psychosocial Oncology, 6*(3/4), 205-216.

Spielberger, C. D., Gorsuch, R. L., & Lushene, R. E. (1970). *STAI manual*. Palo Alto, CA: Consulting Psychologists Press.

Stam, H. J., Koopmans, J. P., & Mathieson, C. M. (1991). The psychosocial impact of laryngectomy: A comprehensive assessment. *Journal of Psychosocial Oncology, 9*(3), 37-58.

Suen, H. K. (1990). *Principles of test theories*. Hillsdale, NJ: Lawrence Erlbaum.

Sutherland, H. J., Lockwood, G. A., & Cunningham, A. J. (1989). A simple, rapid method for assessing psychological distress in cancer patients: Evidence of validity for linear analog scales. *Journal of Psychosocial Oncology, 7*(1/2), 31-43.

Syrjala, K. L., Cummings, C., & Donaldson, G. W. (1992). Hypnosis or cognitive behavioral training for the reduction of pain and nausea during cancer treatment: A controlled clinical trial. *Pain, 48*, 137-146.

Tchekmedyian, N. S., & Cella, D. F. (Eds.). (1990). Quality of life in current oncology practice and research (special issue). *Oncology, 4*(5).

Turpin, G. (Ed.). (1989). *Handbook of clinical psychophysiology.* Plymouth, UK: John Wiley & Sons.

Waligora-Serafin, B., McMahon, T., Pruitt, B. T., & Davenport, J. (1992). Relationships between emotional distress and psychosocial concerns among newly diagnosed cancer patients. *Journal of Psychosocial Oncology, 10*(3), 57-74.

Weisman, A. D., & Worden, J. W. (1976). The existential plight in cancer: Significance of the first 100 days. *International Journal of Psychiatric Medicine, 7,* 1-15.

Weissman, M. M., Sholomskas, D., Pottenger, M., Prusoff, B. A., & Locke, B. Z. (1977). Assessing depressive symptoms in five psychiatric populations: A validation study. *American Journal of Epidemiology, 106,* 203-214.

Wong, C. A., & Bramwell, L. (1992). Uncertainty and anxiety after mastectomy for breast cancer. *Cancer Nursing, 15,* 363-371.

Zabora, J. R., Smith-Wilson, R., Fetting, J. H., & Enterline, J. P. (1990). An efficient method for psychosocial screening of cancer patients. *Psychosomatics, 31,* 192-196.

Zigmond, A. S., & Snaith, R. P. (1983). The Hospital Anxiety and Depression Scale. *Acta Psychiatrica Scandinavica, 67,* 361-370.

Psychosocial Resource Variables in Cancer Research: Statistical and Analytical Considerations

Steven J. Breckler, PhD

SUMMARY. A variety of statistical and analytical issues should be considered whenever psychosocial resource variables are used in cancer research. Measures of resource variables should not be used unless their validity and reliability have been firmly established. Once one decides to measure a resource variable, the sample must be large enough to detect real effects. Most resource variables are measured along a quantitative dimension (e.g., low to high self-esteem). The common practice of imposing cut points on such measures often produces a loss of valuable information. It is also important to recognize that most of the commonly used statistical methods represent only linear relationships among variables. Special statistical methods are needed to represent potential nonlinear relationships. Distinguishing between resource variables that function as moderators and those that function as mediators can be useful. Finally, multivariate statistical methods such as factor analysis and covariance structure modeling provide powerful tools for analyzing psychosocial resource variables, but they must be used with caution. *[Article copies are available from The Haworth Document Delivery Service: 1-800-342-9678.]*

Dr. Breckler is Associate Professor, Department of Psychology, Ames Hall, The Johns Hopkins University, Baltimore, MD 21218. The author wishes to thank Elizabeth C. Wiggins for her comments on an earlier draft of the article.

[Haworth co-indexing entry note]: "Psychosocial Resource Variables in Cancer Research: Statistical and Analytical Considerations." Breckler, Steven J. Co-published simultaneously in the *Journal of Psychosocial Oncology* (The Haworth Medical Press, an imprint of The Haworth Press, Inc.) Vol. 13, No. 1/2, 1995, pp. 161-176; and: *Psychosocial Resource Variables in Cancer Studies: Conceptual and Measurement Issues* (ed: Barbara Curbow, and Mark R. Somerfield), The Haworth Medical Press, an imprint of The Haworth Press, Inc., 1995, pp. 161-176. *[Single or multiple copies of this article are available from The Haworth Document Delivery Service: 1-800-342-9678, 9:00 a.m. - 5:00 p.m. (EST)].*

A variety of statistical and analytical issues should be considered whenever psychosocial resource variables are used in cancer research. This article reviews several such issues, with special reference to problems that arise when measures of individual differences are involved.

TEST CONSTRUCTION, RELIABILITY, AND VALIDITY

Resource variables often represent individual differences in some underlying psychological construct. Examples include self-esteem (Curbow & Somerfield, 1991) and, in this volume, perceived control (Thompson & Collins), religiosity (Jenkins & Pargament), and coping efficacy (Parle & Maguire). Because psychological constructs can never be observed directly, one must rely on one or more instruments or scales to measure the construct of interest. For example, self-esteem can be measured with scales developed by Rosenberg (1965), Hovland and Janis (1959), or Coopersmith (1967), to name just a few (see Wylie, 1974, for descriptions of many other measures of self-esteem).

Measures of psychological constructs are never perfect. One important factor to consider is the *reliability* of an instrument, the degree to which the instrument produces consistent results over time. (See Cronbach, 1990, and Anastasi, 1988, for an overview of reliability assessment; see Allen & Yen, 1979, for details of the underlying theory of measurement.)

Reliability is typically expressed in the form of a correlation coefficient. One approach is to divide the items in an instrument into two subsets or halves, then correlate the scores on the two halves (split-half reliability). A generalization of this approach is to compute *coefficient alpha,* which reflects the internal consistency of multiple items in a test. If the same test is administered twice, the correlation between the two administrations (the test-retest correlation) can also be interpreted as an index of reliability.

Even a perfectly reliable instrument may fail to represent the psychological construct it is intended to measure. Thus, establishing the *validity* of any potential measure of a psychosocial resource variable is important. Like reliability, validity is typically expressed in the form of one or more correlation coefficients. *Convergent validity* is established by showing that the instrument is correlated with other measures of the same underlying construct. *Discriminant validity* is established by showing that the instrument is *not* correlated with measures of other (presumably unrelated) constructs. *Predictive validity* is established by showing that the instrument is correlated with relevant future outcomes.

An instrument should not be used if reliability and validity statistics are not available. Similarly, a newly developed instrument should always be presented with supporting reliability and validity data. Before using a previously developed instrument, one must learn the details surrounding its development. Fresh validation data are generally required whenever a scale is used in a way that deviates from the conditions under which the scale was originally validated. For example, if a scale was originally developed and validated with children, its use with adults is inappropriate unless it has also been validated in adult populations. Curbow and Somerfield (1991) pointed out the diversity of scoring practices that are used with the Rosenberg Self-Esteem Scale (1965). This not only makes comparisons between studies difficult, it also may threaten the validity of the scale.

STATISTICAL POWER ANALYSIS

Individual differences are typically measured in a sample of respondents who have been randomly selected from some population. The typical goal is to make some inference about the population based on the data collected in the sample. Inferential statistics are used for this purpose. Examples include the *t*-test, the *F*-ratio, and the chi-square statistic (see Hays, 1994). Whenever an inferential statistic is used to evaluate a hypothesis, one of two errors is possible. Most data analysts focus on the Type I error, which is the incorrect rejection of a "true" null hypothesis. The likelihood of committing a Type I error (alpha) is set before computing the test statistic, commonly known as the *p*-value. The Type II error, mentioned less often, is the failure to reject a false null hypothesis. The likelihood of committing a Type II error is known as beta. The complement of beta (i.e., 1 minus beta) represents the likelihood of correctly rejecting a false null hypothesis. This quantity also is known as *statistical power* (Cohen, 1977, 1992).

That the data analyst would like as much statistical power as possible should be obvious. At a minimum, one should know how much power accompanies any given statistical test. Power is determined by a number of important factors. Power increases as the probability of a Type I error (alpha) increases. However, increasing power by deliberately increasing alpha is not generally advised.

Power also increases as the size of the effect in the population increases. In correlation units, a small effect corresponds to a correlation of .10; a medium effect, to a correlation of .30; and a large effect, to a correlation of .50 (Cohen, 1977). The true effect size cannot be manipulated, but having some idea or estimate of its magnitude is important. If an empirical estimate of the effect size is unavailable, then a reasonable approach is to estimate its value as the smallest effect that is logically or theoretically relevant.

Power also increases as sample size increases–a design feature that *can* be controlled. Indeed, investigators commonly gain power by adding subjects or respondents to the study.

Statistical power analysis can be used in two distinct ways (Cohen, 1977). First, one can estimate the required sample size given (1) an estimated effect size, (2) the probability of a Type I error, and (3) a desired degree of power. Table 1 illustrates this use of power analysis for detecting a reliable correlation (*r*). The probability of a Type I error of .05 (nondirectional or "two-tailed") is assumed. Nine scenarios are considered; these involve combinations of three estimates of effect size (.10, .30, .50) and three levels of desired power (.70, .80, .90). The sample sizes needed under the nine scenarios vary dramatically. For example, 864 respondents or subjects are needed to detect a small effect (.10) with a high degree of power (.90). In contrast, only 31 respondents are needed to detect a relatively large effect (.50) with the same degree of power. Researchers clearly need to be aware of the size of the effects they wish to study and must adjust their sample sizes accordingly.

The second use of statistical power analysis is to estimate the obtained degree of power given (1) an estimated effect size, (2) a Type I error probability (alpha), and (3) sample size. Table 2 illustrates this use of power analysis for hypotheses involving a correla-

TABLE 1. Illustration of the Required Sample Size, Given Effect Size and Desired Power.[a]

Effect Size	Desired Power	Sample Size Needed
.10	.70	470
.10	.80	618
.10	.90	864
.30	.70	51
.30	.80	68
.30	.90	93
.50	.70	18
.50	.80	22
.50	.90	31

[a]A nondirectional Type I error probability of .05 is assumed. Values are taken from Cohen (1977, Table 3.4.1).

tion coefficient (r). The probability of a Type I error of .05 (nondirectional or two-tailed) is assumed. Nine scenarios are again considered; these involve combinations of three effect size estimates of effect size (.10, .30, .50) and three sample sizes (20, 50, 100). For the small effect size (.10), relatively poor power is obtained even for a sample size of 100. For the moderate effect size (.30), only the largest sample (100) produces acceptable power. For the large effect size (.50), the sample sizes of 50 and 100 both produce high degrees of power. Whenever a nonsignificant correlation is observed, the data analyst should estimate the obtained power to help determine the likelihood of a Type II error.

CUT POINTS IMPOSED ON QUANTITATIVE MEASURES

Many resource variables are measured along a quantitative dimension. For example, most measures of self-esteem produce values that vary along a continuum from low to high. The values produced by such a scale can be used in correlational analyses to determine linear relationships with other input or output variables.

TABLE 2. Illustration of Estimated Power, Given Effect Size and Sample Size.[a]

Effect Size	Sample Size	Estimated Power
.10	20	.11
.10	50	.17
.10	100	.26
.30	20	.37
.30	50	.69
.30	100	.92
.50	20	.75
.50	50	.98
.50	100	> .995

[a] A nondirectional Type I error probability of .05 is assumed. Values are taken from Cohen (1977, Table 3.3.2).

The full observed range of values is generally left intact whenever the measure is treated as a dependent or outcome variable. However, the observed values are sometimes placed into a smaller number of discrete categories, especially when the measure is treated as a predictor or input variable. One common practice is to split observed values at the median. For example, a median split of observed scores on a self-esteem scale would produce two discrete categories, perhaps labeled "low" and "high" self-esteem for values that are below and above the median, respectively.

The practice of imposing cut points on otherwise quantitative measures is generally not recommended. One problem is that the observed range of values in a given sample may not span the entire potential range. If the majority of respondents in a sample score near the high end of the self-esteem continuum, a median split will force half of the respondents into the category labeled "low self-esteem" even though most of them actually score near the high end. More generally, whenever the majority of respondents are clustered at any point along the continuum, a median split introduces artificial variability that is not representative of the sample.

Another problem occurs when the observed range of values in a given sample *does* span the entire potential range. In this case, a median split will cause a loss of information and an attenuation of variability that is truly representative of the sample. The loss of information can have undesired statistical consequences. To illustrate, consider the hypothetical scatter plot of the two quantitative variables shown in Figure 1. The 18 observations exhibit variability along both axes and a strong linear relationship between the two variables. The correlation coefficient (r) for these hypothetical data is .96, with a proportion of shared variability (r^2) of .92. Figure 2 shows the same data, but values along the horizontal axis have been split at the median to form two discrete categories. Clearly, information representing the linear relationship has been lost. Moreover, the correlation coefficient drops to .84 and the proportion of shared variability (r^2) drops to .71.

Data analysts are often motivated to impose cut points so that an otherwise quantitative variable can be treated as a "grouping factor" for purposes of conducting a t-test or analysis of variance (ANOVA). This practice is discouraged because it can lead to misleading conclusions (as described earlier) and because it is unnecessary. Methods of multiple linear regression can accommodate quantitative measures even in combination with truly qualitative or grouping variables (Cohen & Cohen, 1983).

One situation in which cut points are used appropriately is when the instrument does not represent interval information about the construct being measured. As an empirical example, blood donors are often characterized by the extent of their past experience with blood donation. One approach is to use a donor's *number* of previous donations as an indicator of experience. However, this approach assumes that the extent of the donor's psychological experience is a linear function of the actual number of previous donations–an assumption that is probably unwarranted (Piliavin, Evans, & Callero, 1984). Indeed, relatively greater experience is gained from one's first or second donation than from one's fiftiethth donation. Thus, recent studies of the motivation to donate blood have used cut points to classify donors into one of three or four groups that better reflect donors' perceptions of their own previous experience and represent important milestones in the development of a blood do-

FIGURE 1. Scatter Plot of Hypothetical Data that Allows Full Observed Variability on Both Axes.

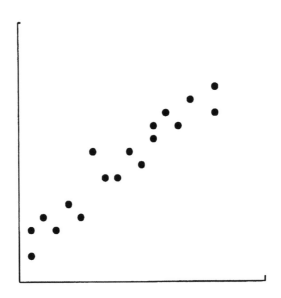

nor's career (Breckler, 1994; Breckler & Wiggins, 1993; Piliavin, Evans, & Callero, 1984).

CORRELATIONS REPRESENT LINEAR RELATIONSHIPS

The general linear model provides the foundation for most of the commonly used statistical methods, including regression, ANOVA, factor analysis, and covariance structure modeling (see Cliff, 1987; Tabachnick & Fidell, 1989). At the heart of these methods is the correlation coefficient or the covariance, both of which are numerical indexes of the extent and direction of a *linear* relationship between two variables.

Concluding that two variables are not related simply because the magnitude of the correlation between them is small may be a mistake. That the two variables do not enjoy a linear association may be true; however, a variety of nonlinear relationships are possible and

FIGURE 2. Scatter Plot of Hypothetical Data, with Observations Dichoto-
mized Below and Above the Median Along the Horizontal Axis.

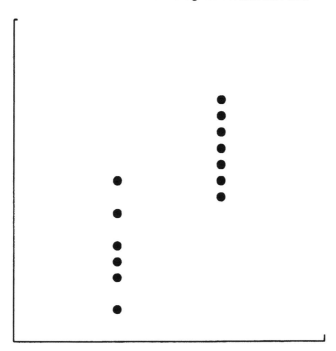

may be functionally important. As a hypothetical example, poor
coping strategies may characterize patients who have either extremely low or extremely high feelings of self-efficacy, whereas
patients who have moderate levels of self-efficacy may exhibit
highly effective coping strategies. The hypothetical relationship
between self-efficacy and coping can therefore be described by an
inverted U-shaped function. The correlation coefficient in this case
could be extremely small, or even zero, even if the two variables are
strongly related.

Psychosocial resource variables may be (and often are) related to
other input or output variables in nonlinear ways. How does the
researcher assess the presence of nonlinear relationships? The best
way is to visualize the data. Bivariate scatter plots can reveal non-
linearities that are often obscured by numerical indexes of associa-

tion such as the correlation coefficient. Once a potential nonlinear relationship has been identified, several data-analytic options are available. For example, multiple linear regression can be used to model certain curvilinear (e.g., quadratic, cubic, quartic) relationships (Cohen & Cohen, 1983). More generally, nonlinear regression procedures are available that can be used to model a large variety of nonlinear relationships.

MODERATORS AND MEDIATORS

Psychosocial resource variables sometimes function as moderators, sometimes as mediators, and sometimes as both. The psychological literature reveals considerable confusion about the difference between moderator variables and mediator variables (Baron & Kenny, 1986; James & Brett, 1984).

A moderator is any variable that influences or modifies the relationship between two other variables. The moderator may strengthen or weaken the relationship, or it may actually change the direction of the relationship. For example, Matt and Dean (1993) found that the relationship between social support from friends and psychological distress was stronger among people older than 70 years than among people between the ages of 50 and 70 years. That is, age was a moderator of the relationship between support and distress. Note that age is not hypothesized as causing the relationship, only as modifying it.

Figure 3 offers a schematic representation of a moderator effect. The moderator variable is assumed to influence the *relationship* between an input variable and an output variable; the moderator is *not* viewed as explaining or causing the relationship. The data-analytic strategy for establishing that a variable functions as a moderator is to examine the *interaction* between the input variable and the candidate moderator (Baron & Kenny, 1986). When two qualitative variables are involved, ANOVA can be used with two main effect terms (the input variable and the moderator variable) and an interaction term representing the moderator effect. When the moderator, the predictor variable, or both are quantitative, analysis of interactions can be done using multiple linear regression with a hierarchical strategy (Baron & Kenny, 1986; Cohen & Cohen, 1983).

FIGURE 3. Schematic Representation of a Moderator Effect.

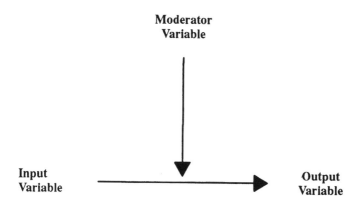

In contrast, a mediator is any variable that accounts for or explains the relationship between two variables. For example, Thompson and Collins (this volume) document the positive relationship that is generally observed between perceptions of personal control and the favorability of outcomes among people who live with a chronic illness. In their article, Thompson and Collins consider several potential mediators (e.g., self-efficacy) that could explain this relationship. That is, self-efficacy may account for the observed relationship between perceptions of control and favorable outcomes. Similarly, Parle and Maguire (this volume) suggest that coping serves as a mediator between the perceived threat of cancer and outcomes such as mental and physical health.

Figure 4 offers a schematic representation of a mediator effect. Here, the mediator is assumed to account for or explain the relationship between the input variable and the output variable. Testing for mediation is not straightforward. Baron and Kenny (1986) recommended a strategy involving three regression equations. In the first equation, a simple linear regression analysis must show that the input variable is a reliable predictor of the mediator (Path a). In the second equation, a simple linear regression analysis must show that the input variable is a reliable predictor of the output variable (Path c). In the third equation, a multiple linear regression analysis must show that the mediator is a reliable predictor of the output variable

FIGURE 4. Schematic Representation of a Mediator Effect.

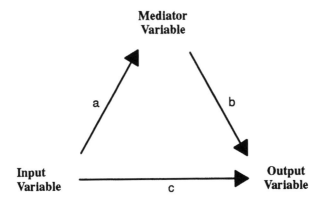

(Path b) when the equation also includes the input variable as a predictor. Under these conditions, mediation is established if the correlation observed between the input and output variables (Path c) is diminished, or even vanishes, when the candidate mediator variable is partialed.

' MULTIVARIATE STATISTICAL CONSIDERATIONS

A variety of multivariate statistical methods are used to analyze measures of psychosocial resource variables. For example, multi-item scales are often subjected to factor analysis (Gorsuch, 1983) to help identify potential subcomponents of the scale. The results of a single factor analysis, however, should be interpreted with caution. In the case of exploratory factor analysis, for example, the interpretation of factors is necessarily a post hoc endeavor. Once a factor model is developed, new data should be collected to validate the initial interpretation. Confirmatory factor analysis (Long, 1983a) provides an especially powerful tool for such cross-validation studies.

Methods of covariance structure modeling (Hayduk, 1987; Loehlin, 1987; Long, 1983b) have become popular for analyzing relationships between psychosocial resource variables and various input and output variables (e.g., Matt & Dean, 1993). These methods merge the logic of confirmatory factor analysis, multiple regression, and path analysis within a single data-analytic framework. Among the many applications are estimation of disattenuated correlation and regression coefficients, evaluation of multitrait-multimethod matrices, and assessment of hypothesized causal structures. Shortcomings of these methods are commonly acknowledged in the mathematical literature and in textbooks. Nevertheless, users of these methods often fail to recognize the potential problems (for help in identifying such problems, see Breckler, 1990; Cliff, 1983; or MacCallum, 1986). For example, the fact that the fit of a particular, favored model is identical for a potentially large family of "equivalent" models (Stelzl, 1986) is rarely acknowledged. Researchers also tend to rely on covariance structure modeling to support causal inferences even though the data analytic method, by itself, does not provide a sufficient basis for inferring causation.

Obtaining a sufficient sample size is a special problem when multivariate data sets are involved (see Harris, 1985). Small samples can produce unreliable parameter estimates and results that fail to replicate in new samples. Although firm guidelines for determining the appropriate sample size cannot be given, several informal rules can be helpful. For example, some data analysts focus on the ratio of respondents to measured variables. At a minimum, this ratio should be 10:1, with ratios of 20:1 or greater generally being preferred. This means that a factor analysis involving 40 measured variables should be based on a *minimum* sample size of 400, preferably on a sample size of 800 or more.

Unstable results can be expected when the sample size is too small. In the case of correlation and regression analyses, the magnitude, and even the sign, of regression coefficients can change from sample to sample. Factor analyses that are based on small samples can produce unreliable factor loadings and nonreplicable or spurious factors. Large samples are typically required for proper estimation of covariance structure models (Tanaka, 1987).

Small samples are often unavoidable, especially in applied research settings. If the goal is to develop a new measure of individual difference, resources must be marshalled to ensure that the sample size is sufficient to establish the reliability and validity of the instrument. However, if the goal is to apply a previously developed instrument, smaller sample sizes can be tolerated. In these cases, the researcher must anticipate reduced sensitivity to interventions or treatments and recognize the potential threats to valid inference. For example, factor structures that were found when an instrument was originally developed may not be observed when it is used with a smaller sample.

CONCLUSION

Psychosocial resource variables present a variety of statistical and analytical challenges, some of which have been briefly discussed in this article. The measurement of psychosocial resource variables demands attention to issues of reliability and validity. Establishing the direction and magnitude of interventions requires careful consideration of statistical power and sample size. The common practice of imposing cut points on otherwise quantitative variables can introduce serious artifacts. Linear statistical methods such as multiple regression may obscure important nonlinear relationships. Special analytical approaches are needed to establish psychosocial resource variables as mediators or moderators. Elaborate multivariate statistical methods can be helpful, but they must be used with caution.

It is hoped that this review will help investigators avoid statistical and analytical problems in their treatment of psychosocial resource variables. Perhaps it suggests new approaches to the study of individual differences in adjustment to cancer and cancer treatment.

REFERENCES

Allen, M. J., & Yen, W. M. (1979). *Introduction to measurement theory.* Monterey, CA: Brooks/Cole.

Anastasi, A. (1988). *Psychological testing* (6th ed.). New York: Macmillan.

Baron, R. M., & Kenny, D. A. (1986). The moderator-mediator variable distinction in social psychological research: Conceptual, strategic, and statistical considerations. *Journal of Personality & Social Psychology, 51,* 1173-1182.

Breckler, S. J. (1990). Applications of covariance structure modeling in psychology: Cause for concern? *Psychological Bulletin, 107,* 260-273.

Breckler, S. J. (1994). Memory for the experience of donating blood: Just how bad was it? *Basic & Applied Social Psychology, 15,* 467-488.

Breckler, S. J., & Wiggins, E. C. (1993). Emotional responses and the affective component of attitude. *Journal of Social Behavior & Personality, 8,* 281-296.

Cliff, N. (1983). Some cautions concerning the application of causal modeling methods. *Multivariate Behavioral Research, 18,* 115-126.

Cliff, N. (1987). *Analyzing multivariate data.* San Diego, CA: Harcourt Brace Jovanovich.

Cohen, J. (1977). *Statistical power analysis for the behavioral sciences* (rev. ed.). New York: Academic Press.

Cohen, J. (1992). A power primer. *Psychological Bulletin, 112,* 155-159.

Cohen, J., & Cohen, P. (1983). *Applied multiple regression/correlation analysis for the behavioral sciences* (2nd ed.). Hillsdale, NJ: Lawrence Erlbaum.

Coopersmith, S. (1967). *The antecedents of self-esteem.* San Francisco, CA: W. H. Freeman.

Cronbach, L. J. (1990). *Essentials of psychological testing.* New York: Harper & Row.

Curbow, B., & Somerfield, M. (1991). Use of the Rosenberg Self-Esteem Scale with adult cancer patients. *Journal of Psychosocial Oncology, 9*(2), 113-131.

Gorsuch, R. L. (1983). *Factor analysis* (2nd ed.). Hillsdale, NJ: Lawrence Erlbaum.

Harris, R. J. (1985). *A primer of multivariate statistics* (2nd ed.). Orlando, FL: Academic Press.

Hayduk, L. A. (1987). *Structural equation modeling with LISREL.* Baltimore, MD: Johns Hopkins University Press.

Hays, W. L. (1994). *Statistics* (5th ed.). Fort Worth, TX: Harcourt Brace Jovanovich.

Hovland, C. I., & Janis, I. (Eds). (1959). *Personality and persuasibility.* New Haven, CT: Yale University Press.

James, L. R., & Brett, J. M. (1984). Mediators, moderators, and tests for mediation. *Journal of Applied Psychology, 69,* 307-321.

Loehlin, J. C. (1987). *Latent variable models: An introduction to factor, path, and structural analysis.* Hillsdale, NJ: Lawrence Erlbaum.

Long, J. S. (1983a). *Confirmatory factor analysis.* Beverly Hills, CA: Sage Publications.

Long, J. S. (1983b). *Covariance structure models: An introduction to LISREL.* Beverly Hills, CA: Sage Publications.

MacCallum, R. (1986). Specification searches in covariance structure modeling. *Psychological Bulletin, 100,* 107-120.

Matt, G. E., & Dean, A. (1993). Social support from friends and psychological distress among elderly persons: Moderator effects of age. *Journal of Health & Social Behavior, 34,* 187-200.

Piliavin, J. A., Evans, D. E., & Callero, P. L. (1984). Learning to give to unnamed strangers: The process of commitment to regular blood donation. In E. Staub, D. Bar-Tal, J. Karylowski, & J. Reykowski (Eds.), *The development and maintenance of prosocial behavior: International perspectives* (pp. 471-492). New York: Plenum Press.

Rosenberg, M. (1965). *Society and the adolescent self-image*. Princeton, NJ: Princeton University Press.

Stelzl, I. (1986). Changing a causal hypothesis without changing the fit: Some rules for generating equivalent path models. *Multivariate Behavioral Research, 21*, 309-331.

Tabachnick, B. G., & Fidell, L. S. (1989). *Using multivariate statistics*. New York: Harper-Collins.

Tanaka, J. S. (1987). "How big is big enough?": Sample size and goodness of fit in structural equation models with latent variables. *Child Development, 58*, 134-146.

Wylie, R. C. (1974). *The self-concept* (Vol. 1). Lincoln: University of Nebraska Press.

The Use of Qualitative Methods to Strengthen Psychosocial Research on Cancer

Nancy Waxler-Morrison, PhD
Richard Doll, MSW, MSc
T. Gregory Hislop, MDCM

SUMMARY. Most research on psychosocial issues in cancer follows a quantitative strategy, using standard instruments and statistical analyses, yet researchers sometimes pay less attention to matters of validity. The authors propose a research strategy that combines qualitative and quantitative methods. The qualitative method is used to discover variables and define hypotheses and thus strengthen validity, and quantitative techniques are used to establish statistical significance and thus generalizability. The usefulness of the strategy is illustrated with examples from noncancer and cancer research, and some practical issues concerning the use of the less familiar qualitative techniques are discussed. *[Article copies are available from The Haworth Document Delivery Service: 1-800-342-9678.]*

Dr. Waxler-Morrison is Associate Professor Emerita, Department of Anthropology and Sociology, University of British Columbia, Vancouver, British Columbia, Canada. Mr. Doll is Chair and Head, Patient and Family Counselling, and Dr. Hislop is Senior Epidemiologist, Division of Epidemiology, Biometry and Occupational Oncology, British Columbia Cancer Agency, Vancouver. (Address correspondence to Mr. Doll, Patient and Family Counselling, British Columbia Cancer Agency, 600 West 10th Avenue, Vancouver, BC, Canada V5Z 4E6.)

[Haworth co-indexing entry note]: "The Use of Qualitative Methods to Strengthen Psychosocial Research on Cancer." Waxler-Morrison, Nancy, Richard Doll, and T. Gregory Hislop. Co-published simultaneously in the *Journal of Psychosocial Oncology* (The Haworth Medical Press, an imprint of The Haworth Press, Inc.) Vol. 13, No. 1/2, 1995, pp. 177-191; and: *Psychosocial Resource Variables in Cancer Studies: Conceptual and Measurement Issues* (ed: Barbara Curbow, and Mark R. Somerfield), The Haworth Medical Press, an imprint of The Haworth Press, Inc., 1995, pp. 177-191. *[Single or multiple copies of this article are available from The Haworth Document Delivery Service: 1-800-342-9678, 9:00 a.m. - 5:00 p.m. (EST)].*

One only needs to skim through articles in this journal and similar journals to see that research using structured interviews, standard scales, and systematic questionnaires that produce data in quantitative form is the most common approach to investigating and reporting on psychosocial factors in cancer. However, in an effort to meet such scientific standards as objectivity and the use of statistical tests to rule out chance observations, we may sometimes give short shrift to the more difficult problem of validity. Are we certain we are measuring the most important variables and testing the most relevant hypotheses–that is, are we producing data that accurately represent the phenomena of interest?

Jenkins and Pargament (this volume) raise this question when discussing measures of religion as a technique for coping with illness. Many surveys include one or two closed-ended questions, often on religious membership or attendance, and many respondents answer both questions in the negative. As a result, we often conclude that religion as a coping technique is not significant. Yet, when one gives the respondent an opportunity to speak freely about religion in his or her life, as Jenkins (1985) did, one finds that people who do not identify with organized religion do indeed use religious coping mechanisms and view religion as important. Those of us who have used the "standard" questions may have been asking the wrong questions and producing invalid information.

This article describes a research strategy that explicitly deals with problems of validity but does not lose the strength of statistical testing and generalization. For example, in this strategy, qualitative techniques, unstructured ethnographic interviews of cancer patients or participant observations of support groups are used initially to discover important variables and develop hypotheses. These variables are then measured and hypotheses are statistically tested in subsequent quantitative research such as an epidemiological study using a structured questionnaire.

The combination of qualitative and quantitative methods is certainly not new to social science and medicine. The strategy is sometimes used by social demographers, social epidemiologists, and medical anthropologists; however, the approach is not common in psychosocial research on cancer. Therefore, after briefly discussing the underlying assumptions of quantitative and qualitative methods, we will present research examples that have used the strategy to improve validity and discuss some practical issues involved in doing the less familiar qualitative work.

STRENGTHS AND WEAKNESSES OF THE METHODS

Qualitative and quantitative research methods rest on two different ways of knowing; each has its own philosophical base, methodological concerns, and research strategies, and each, of course, has many subtypes or variations. The strategy discussed here, in which qualitative methods are used to discover hypotheses that are later tested quantitatively, is only one of the many uses of the qualitative technique. Some researchers argue that it is unnecessary or impossible to combine the methods, given that they are based on different theories (Rubenstein & Perloff, 1986). (For interesting discussions of some of these issues, see Janes, Stall, & Gifford; Silverman, 1993; Tebes & Kraemer, 1991). From the particular perspective of this article, quantitative research usually involves deductive reasoning, with a primary focus on hypothesis testing of phenomena that are counted and compared. On the other hand, qualitative research usually uses unstructured data collection methods and involves inductive reasoning to develop hypotheses and to understand the complexity and meaning of experience presented in the form of themes.

Quantitative research methods provide systematic measures of specified variables for all subjects and thus allow the comparison of these variables across subgroups within the study test hypotheses. When combined with random sampling, statistical tests can be used and the findings can be generalized to a larger population. Findings also can be compared with those of similar studies to help establish the importance of the observations. Data are often collected in the form of personal interviews or questionnaires using precoded questions, but the same techniques can be applied to the coding of hospital charts or of group process, for example. From our viewpoint, a major limitation of such methods is that one cannot discover new or unexpected variables: that is, factors beyond those that were measured. In fact, the variables measured may be the unimportant ones. If this is true, even with the addition of elegant statistical methods, one would never be able to provide a full and valid picture of the phenomena of interest.

Qualitative methods are often used to understand a person's experience from his or her own point of view, sometimes by using an unstructured ethnographic interview . . . in which people are encouraged to tell their stories in any way they choose. Techniques of qualitative analysis also can be applied to data collected by participant observations, to written records, to transcripts of group discussions, and to open-ended questions inserted in structured questionnaires. Because the purpose is discovery, not verification, sample sizes are often small and samples are nonrandom. Although a number of data analysis strategies are available (and will be discussed later), investigators usually immerse themselves in the raw data and use inductive thinking to discover common themes and variables and to develop hypotheses (Strauss & Corbin, 1990). A great strength of such qualitative methods is the opportunity to discover new hypotheses and variables. A limitation is that one cannot obtain comparable data from all subjects; hence, groups of subjects cannot be compared.

UNDERSTANDING OF NON-CANCER-RELATED ILLNESS

The benefits of combining qualitative methods with quantitative methods have been demonstrated in investigations of a number of health and illness issues. We will discuss two of these studies in some detail to demonstrate the advantages of this strategy.

Janes (1986) began with quantitative survey data, moved to a qualitative study to identify crucial variables and hypotheses, then returned to a quantitative study to test these new hypotheses. The epidemiological research of Janes and others suggested that Samoans who had migrated to the United States experienced significant increases in both weight and blood pressure. However, these epidemiological studies showed that the usual explanations for changes in migrants–that is, changes in diet–accounted for only a small proportion of the variation. Furthermore, these studies reported unexplained differences between Samoan men and women. Clearly, qualitative methods could be useful to provide specific information about the stresses of migration and how these are experienced by different members of the Samoan community.

Janes's qualitative techniques consisted of standard anthropological ethnographic methods, including observing and informally interviewing members of a Samoan community centered on a large church in Los Angeles. New and specific factors that may link migration to obesity or high blood pressure were uncovered with this method. For example, when Samoans move to the United States, they leave an economy in which most people have the security of land to an economy that requires jobs and money. Many must take low-income jobs, which means they are unable to maintain the family's prestige and status, particularly through generous and expensive rituals such as weddings and contributions to the church, the center of Samoan life. The resulting conflict between providing for one's family and participating in the church is especially difficult for the older women, who are expected to be family and church leaders.

Janes's qualitative methods were extremely fruitful and thus allowed him to move to the third quantitative stage, a survey of a representative sample of 115 adults. Following from his qualitative findings, Janes asked about family income, leadership in the community, and participation in important rituals. He then measured the respondents' blood pressure and weight and found, for example, that Samoans who had low incomes but participated frequently in rituals, and hence experienced more conflict or stress, had significantly higher blood pressure than did those who had higher incomes and participated frequently in rituals. Furthermore, this effect was much stronger for women. Thus, by using qualitative methods to understand the specific experiences of Samoan immigrants, the explanatory links between migration and blood pressure were specified much more clearly, and these associations were validated in a quantitative study with a large sample. Diet disappeared from the model and, instead, increased blood pressure was linked to the stress resulting from conflicting social expectations.

Similar research strategies have been used to investigate infant mortality rates in Brazil (Nations & Amaral, 1991), use of immunization programs in Haiti (Coreil et al., 1989), and changes in the use of alcohol as men age (Stall, 1986). Other examples and discussions of methods can be found in Janes, Stall, and Gifford (1986).

UNDERSTANDING PSYCHOSOCIAL FACTORS IN CANCER

Although there are many examples of quantitative research on the psychosocial issues in cancer and a few examples of qualitative studies, few studies have taken advantage of the combination of methods. For example, in our survey of recent issues of the *Journal of Psychosocial Oncology*, we found many studies that used quantitative interviews, tests, and questionnaires; a few that used open-ended interviews, for example, "to help interpret the findings" (Bauman, Gervey, & Siegel, 1992, p. 8); but none that used a qualitative study as a hypothesis-generating technique.

The qualitative studies of cancer that do exist, found more often in the social science literature, demonstrate the usefulness of qualitative methods and could also serve as sources of hypotheses and concepts that could be quantified by others. For example, Maher's exploratory interviews (1982) with recovered cancer patients uncovered often unexpected but perhaps common responses to recovery. These included feeling depressed at the very time one realizes treatment has been successful, being unable to plan for the future, and delaying the expression of anger about the experience of treatment. Clarke's qualitative-type interviews with women (1984) alert us to the changes and problems in relationships with husbands when wives are diagnosed with cancer. (See, also, the qualitative research by Gifford, 1986, & Taylor, 1988.)

To demonstrate the usefulness of the qualitative-quantitative research strategy for understanding the cancer experience, we will now review two of our own studies. In our prognostic study of breast cancer patients (Waxler-Morrison et al., 1991), we began with a large epidemiological survey that was followed, in the second phase, by a small qualitative study. In the first phase, we mailed a questionnaire to a large cohort of women soon after their breast cancer diagnosis had been made. For example, closed-ended generic questions on social support and social networks were taken from the work of others and, in some cases, suitably revised. Data from the sample of 133 women were analyzed at the four-year follow-up period and, using multivariate methods controlling for clinical factors obtained from the women's medical records, we found that women who were more likely to survive had more supportive friends, more contact with friends, and larger social networks; were employed; and were single, divorced, or widowed.

The findings from this quantitative work raised many questions that we could not answer. How might social factors, such as work and friendship, affect survival, if they do? As is often the case with epidemiological studies, the questionnaire provided few additional variables that were useful for investigating these findings; therefore, we moved to a set of open-ended ethnographic interviews with some of the survivors who provided rich descriptive information that might help us understand what the quantitative findings meant.

At the beginning of each interview, the woman was asked to tell us about her cancer experience. The interviewer asked the woman about her work, relationship with friends, social support, and family only if she did not mention them voluntarily. Qualitative analysis of taped interviews produced many hypotheses about the findings from the survey. For example, having a job may be helpful because women tend to work with other women and a co-worker with breast cancer often becomes the center of a large network of information and support. New hypotheses were raised as well, particularly the idea that survival may be linked to the giving of support rather than to simply receiving support. Many of the survivors actively initiated the giving of help to others. These qualitative interviews told us much we had not known about women's experiences with breast cancer; thus, they allowed us to think much more specifically about the associations between the significant social variables and survival.

Following Janes's strategy, we then used the qualitative research information to inform variables measured in a subsequent quantitative study of cancer patients' survival (Doll, Hislop, & Waxler-Morrison, 1987). For example, we have moved beyond generic measures of work experience to include more specific questions about co-workers, their knowledge of the person's cancer diagnosis, and whether they gave help or information.

Having discovered the usefulness of the qualitative-quantitative strategy, we have been using it to study another psychosocial issue in cancer. We began with qualitative methods and used these data to define variables and hypotheses for the second phase, a quantitative study of a large representative sample. The focus of that study of breast cancer survivors (Waxler-Morrison et al., 1992) was understanding the experiences of women who had been successfully treated one, three, or five years earlier. Did they have difficulties returning to their normal roles? If so, did these problems arise in a predictable sequence?

The initial qualitative phase of this research began with interviews of 30 women who had completed treatment for breast cancer, had a good prognosis, had no recurrence, and had completed treatment one, three, or five years earlier. Experienced interviewers opened the interview with a general question: "We might start with the time when you were diagnosed. Could you tell me about that?" The invitation to tell one's story is generally enough to elicit detailed experiences during the entire survival period. Only if areas of special interest to us–work, friendship, family, and relationships with treatment staff–were not mentioned did the interviewer ask other direct questions. Interviews lasted an average of 90 minutes, were taped, and were fully transcribed, producing typescripts averaging 56 pages in length. The use of standard methods of qualitative analysis (Strauss & Corbin, 1990) produced 16 themes that were common to survivors' experiences. These themes were used to code the typescripts and to identify (by reading coded sections of interviews) how, for example, survival issues change across time or vary from older to younger women.

These extremely rich interviews opened up many aspects of the experience of surviving breast cancer that were not prominent in the literature on survival. For example, the experience of having breast cancer and being treated successfully appears to be different for older women (especially those older than 60 years) than it is for younger women (especially those younger than 50 years). For older women, having breast cancer may be distressing and unsettling, but it appears to be a fairly minor crisis in a life containing a major crisis such as a husband's death, illness, or retirement or a child's divorce. For these women, breast cancer often is not nearly as debilitating or worrisome as arthritis or other disabilities. For younger women, the stresses of breast cancer and the difficulties of survival appear to be greater; they are centered on worries about recurrence and on concern about the welfare of their husband and children.

We found two techniques of coping with cancer and fears of recurrence that are not often reported in the literature. Some women become involved in political and lobbying activities, seeking more research and services for breast cancer. They see these activities, at least in part, as a way to handle their own anxiety about cancer. A second, even more common coping technique is represented by survivors who quickly become informal counselors for other women with breast cancer–an activity that is entirely unrelated to formal services. These women report that helping others is a way to "help oneself feel normal again."

The qualitative phase of our study has been invaluable in the second, quantitative phase. We are designing a survey of a representative sample of breast cancer survivors using open- and closed-ended interview questions that can be quantified and statistically analyzed to document the problems of survivors and the sequence in which the problems occur. Specific questions used in this interview are being developed from the qualitative data and are being designed to test some of the hypotheses from those data. For example, to test the hypothesis about age differences in the importance of cancer, we will ask about other noncancer-related life events and life problems that have occurred since the diagnosis and about their importance relative to cancer. To document the informal support system, we will ask whether women sought out other survivors for help and whether others sought them out.

Although the study is not yet complete, it seems clear that the qualitative phase of the work has been crucial in identifying important variables and hypotheses specific to the breast cancer survivor's experience–factors that we would not otherwise have chosen to measure.

PRACTICAL ISSUES

Sampling

When qualitative methods are used as an hypothesis-generating technique, as proposed here, formal random sampling techniques are neither appropriate nor necessary because generalizing from a sample to a larger population is not the goal. However, most researchers do follow certain informal sampling strategies to allow for variation in the data and thus stronger and more general hypotheses. Using the literature and one's knowledge of the topic, one selects a "sample" that encompasses the range of variables one thinks might be important to the issue.

Because the literature suggested that survival issues might change over time, we chose women who had completed treatment one, three, or five years earlier. To represent most women who have breast cancer, we included women ranging in age from 20 through 79 years. (We assumed that most women older than 80 have different survival problems.) To ensure variation in social class, the women's homes were scattered geographically. We assumed that within this group of women of varied length of survival, age, and social class, we would see the broadest range of survival experiences. A similar logic of selection can be followed in any qualitative research with the goal of generating hypotheses.

Analysis

Qualitative data can be analyzed and presented in a variety of ways, each of which is linked to an underlying research philosophy. For example, some anthropologists argue that qualitative data should be presented in their most complete form, without summary, coding, or other intervention by the researcher (Rubinstein & Perloff, 1986). However, the most commonly used analytic method, and the one most useful for generating hypotheses and variables, is based in Strauss's grounded theory approach. In this technique, theory is developed inductively from qualitative analyses of the phenomena of interest (Glaser & Strauss, 1967; Silverman, 1993; Strauss & Corbin, 1990).

Although highly sophisticated ways of analyzing qualitative data are available (Willms et al., 1990), a fairly straightforward and simple method is often suitable. For example, in our study, raw data were in the form of typed interviews. In the first stage, two researchers simply read these interviews to become familiar with the data. Next, they selected a random sample of 10 interviews (out of 30), read them independently, and noted in the margins the topics that the women mentioned (e.g., "problems with job supervisor as result of cancer" or "useful way to cope with chemotherapy"). In the next stage, these topics were jointly reviewed, and many were grouped into more abstract themes (e.g., "prayer" and "changed diet" become specific examples of "coping techniques"). This step produced 16 themes; theme numbers were recorded in the margins of all 30 interviews to allow for quick identification of content. Throughout this process, each researcher made notes on tentative hypotheses, interesting content, and important variables.

One hypothesis involved age differences in the survival experience. To investigate these ideas further, interviews were separated into three age groups. The researchers independently read content from important themes (e.g., fear of death, family relations), discussed the patterns, and agreed on age-related hypotheses to be tested in the quantitative stage of the research.

Computer programs developed for qualitative analysis (e.g., Ethnograph, NUDIST, QUALPRO) (as discussed by Silverman, 1993) can sometimes save analysis time because all identified themes can be recorded directly on the computerized data text. Data that is relevant to any particular theme or subtheme can then be retrieved and reviewed. Our experience suggests that computerized coding and retrieval is more useful with large samples than with small ones. In no way does computerization save the time needed to read, discuss, and think about the qualitative data.

Cost

Researchers are sometimes hesitant to use qualitative methods because they are thought to be costly, which is indeed often true if one simply looks at the cost per subject. Using our breast cancer survivor study as an example, we interviewed 30 women. The total budget for the study was $37,000 (Canadian); therefore, the cost per subject was $1,230. Many qualitative studies are done for much less, especially if transcribing of tapes and travel are not involved. The total budgets of most qualitative studies are small, however, compared with total budgets of many survey or epidemiological studies, which are often three or four times as costly. By combining research strategies, the costs of the qualitative phase are probably outweighed by later benefits, when one can avoid dead-end data analyses and the need for further data collection to follow up on unexplainable or confusing findings.

A hidden cost of qualitative research should be recognized, however. Data analysis, the stage at which data are reviewed, themes are defined, and hypotheses are developed, must be done by a person who is familiar with the literature and the research issues; this person is usually a senior investigator. These analyses are time consuming, but they cannot be handed over easily to a research assistant. (See Willms et al., 1990, for ways of handling this problem.) The same is true of other qualitative data collection techniques, particularly participant observation, which is probably most fruitful if done by a senior investigator.

DISCUSSION

We have argued that research on psychosocial aspects of cancer can be strengthened by using a strategy that combines qualitative and quantitative methods. The qualitative phase of the work serves to identify variables and new hypotheses, often improving validity, whereas the quantitative phase provides for statistical tests and thus generalizability.

The usefulness of this research model is not limited to studies of quality-of-life or adjustment-to-cancer issues. As Janes's study (1986) of high blood pressure in Samoans showed, the exploratory qualitative techniques were crucial in shifting the causal model for hypertension from change in diet to increased social stress. The research strategy may be just as useful to cancer epidemiologists and clinical investigators who are working on causation and treatment.

Why is the research strategy, the qualitative technique in particular, not commonly used to study cancer? We can suggest several reasons. First, biomedical principles are based in quantitative research and physicians are largely trained in these methods. There is little or no understanding of the value and scope of qualitative research. Although physicians may believe that qualitative research is interesting or possibly useful for quality-of-life issues, they often judge it to be of limited value because it has not been applied often to such issues as potential causes or cures of cancer.

Second, social scientists themselves may be partially responsible for the bias toward quantitative research. A reluctance to apply qualitative research techniques that have developed from within their own disciplines may have resulted from a desire to gain acceptance and credibility from physicians and granting bodies (Foster, 1987).

Third, within some cancer organizations, certainly those in Canada, budgets for research often tend to be heavily weighted toward clinical medicine and basic sciences, which have traditionally valued quantitative methods. Only recently have social science researchers, who are more likely to be trained in and to use qualitative techniques, gained significant representation on some grant review committees and thus been able to introduce and support alternative methodologies (Foster, 1987).

All of these factors are in the process of change. The growing patient movement in both the United States and Canada has focused cancer patients' interests on quality of life, involvement in treatment decisions, and "caring versus curing." At the same time, there has been a lack of progress in the cure and control. These factors have led to a shift in relative power of patient and physician that has opened the way to potential changes in research. Social scientists and patient interest groups are now encouraging funding bodies involved in oncology research to give greater consideration to qualitative research, in part so that patients' opinions and experiences can be heard.

Finally, the potential for prognostically important psychosocial interventions may lead to significant shifts in methods of cancer research. The replication of work by Spiegel et al. (1989) in several Canadian cancer centers demonstrates the importance of interdisciplinary research. Oncologists and social researchers have been brought into partnership in areas where, in some cases, little collaboration previously existed. This is just one example of the increasing legitimation of interdisciplinary research that opens up more opportunities for a variety of theoretical and methodological approaches to cancer. The research strategy we propose here may therefore be timely because it can serve as a useful middle ground, one that provides an acceptable methodology to both physicians and social scientists.

REFERENCES

Bauman, L., Gervey, R., & Siegel, K. (1992). Factors associated with cancer patients' participation in support groups. *Journal of Psychosocial Oncology, 10*(3), 1-20.

Clarke, J. (1984). *It's cancer: The personal experiences of women who have received a cancer diagnosis.* Toronto, Ontario, Canada: IPI Publishing.

Coreil, J., Augustin, A., Holt, E., & Halsey, N. (1989). Use of ethnographic research for instrument development in a case-control study of immunization use in Haiti. *International Journal of Epidemiology, 19*(4, Suppl. 2), S33-S37.

Doll, R., Hislop, T. G., & Waxler-Morrison, N. (1987). Prognostic study of social situations and personal attitudes in cancer. Unpublished study, British Columbia Cancer Agency, Vancouver, BC, Canada.

Foster, G. M. (1987). World Health Organization behavioural science research: Problems and prospects. *Social Science & Medicine, 24*, 709-717.

Gifford, S. (1986). The meaning of lumps: A cast study of the ambiguity of risk. In C. Janes, R. Stall, & S. Gifford (Eds.), *Anthropology and epidemiology* (pp. 213-246). Dordrecht, Netherlands: Reidel.

Glaser, B., & Strauss, A. (1967). *The discovery of grounded theory: Strategies for qualitative research.* Chicago: Aldine.

Janes, C. (1986). Migration and hypertension: An ethnography of disease risk in an urban Samoan community. In C. Janes, R. Stall, & S. Gifford (Eds.), *Anthropology and epidemiology* (pp. 175-211). Dordrecht, Netherlands: Reidel.

Janes, C., Stall, R., & Gifford, S. (1986). *Anthropology and epidemiology.* Dordrecht, Netherlands: Reidel.

Jenkins, R. (1985). *An investigation of cognitive attributes of coping in medical patients.* Unpublished doctoral dissertation, Bowling Green State University, Bowling Green, OH.

Maher, E. (1982). Anomic aspects of recovery from cancer. *Social Science & Medicine, 16*, 907-912.

Nations, M., & Amaral, M. (1991). Flesh, blood, souls and households: Cultural validity in mortality inquiry. *Medical Anthropology Quarterly, 5*, 204-219.

Rubinstein, R., & Perloff, J. (1986). Identifying psychosocial disorders in children: On integrating epidemiological and anthropological understandings. In C. Janes, R. Stall, & S. Gifford (Eds.), *Anthropology and epidemiology* (pp. 303-332). Dordrecht, Netherlands: Reidel.

Silverman, D. (1993). *Interpreting qualitative data: Methods for analyzing talk, text and interaction.* Thousand Oaks, CA: Sage Publications.

Spiegel, D., Bloom, J. R., Kraemer, H. C., & Gottheil, E. (1989, October 14). The beneficial effect of psychosocial treatment on survival of metastatic breast cancer patients. *Lancet*, 888-891.

Stall, R. (1986). Respondent-identified reasons for change and stability in alcohol consumption as a concomitant of the aging process. In C. Janes, R. Stall, & S. Gifford (Eds.), *Anthropology and epidemiology* (pp. 275-302). Dordrecht, Netherlands: Reidel.

Strauss, A., & Corbin, J. (1990). *Basics of qualitative research: Grounded theory procedures and techniques.* Newbury Park, CA: Sage Publications.

Taylor, K. (1988). Physicians and the disclosure of undesirable information. In M. Lock & D. Gordon (Eds.), *Biomedicine examined* (pp. 441-463). Dordrecht, Netherlands: Reidel.

Tebes, J., & Kraemer, D. (1991). Quantitative and qualitative knowing in mutual support rsearch: Some lesions from recent history of scientific psychology. *American Journal of Community Psychology, 19*, 739-756.

Waxler-Morrison, N., Hislop, T. G., Mears, B., & Kan, L. (1991). Effects of social relationships on survival for women with breast cancer: A prospective study. *Social Science & Medicine, 3*, 177-183.

Waxler-Morrison, N., Hislop, T. G., & Doll, R. (1992). Cancer survivorship: The psychosocial experiences in breast cancer. Unpublished study, British Columbia Cancer Agency, Vancouver, BC, Canada.

Willms, D., Best, J., Taylor, D., Gilbert, J., Wilson, D., Lindsay, E., & Singer, J. (1990). A systematic approach for using qualitative methods in primary prevention research. *Medical Anthropology Quarterly, 4*, 391-409.

Index

Abrams, M.R., 55
Abramson, L.Y., 13,15
Achterberg-Lawlis, J., 56,60
Acklin, M.W., 56,60
Adaptability vs. flexibility, 100
Adaptation
  active vs. passive, 3-4
  direct (main) effects model, 5-6
  immune model, 3
  religious/spiritual
  mechanisms of, 56-63
  self-management and, 63-84
  resistance perspective, 3-4
  social support and, 79-86
  vulnerability perspective, 3
Adelman, M.B., 76,78,92
Adult Nowicki-Strickland
      Internal-External Control
      Scale (ANSIE), 16-17
Affective disorders, 44,46. See also
      Anxiety; Depression
Affects Balance Scale (Derogatis),
      143
Affleck, G.,13
African-American
  social support studies, 104
African-Americans
  and religion/spirituality, 59
Age
  and perceived control, 20
  and religion/spirituality, 59-60
  social support and psychological
      distress in elderly, 77-78
AIDS
  and perceived control, 21-22
  and religious coping, 67
Albany Medical College, 75-92
Albrecht, T.L., 75-92,76,77,78,92

Aldwin, C.M., 29
Allen, M.J., 162
Alloy, L.B., 15
Allport, G.W., 60
Alvarez, W., 142
Amaral, M., 181
Amelioration vs. prevention, 4-5
American Cancer Society, 98,124
American Cancer Society Workshop,
      124
American Indians. See Native
      Americans
Amish studies, 101
Analytical issues, 161-175. See also
      Statistical/analytical issues
Anastasi, A., 19,137,162
Anderson, J., 132,134,136,140,141
Angel, R., 148
Angell, R., 99
Anger and outcome, 41-42
Animal behavioral studies, 30-31
ANOVA (analysis of variance),
      167,170
ANSIE (Adult Nowicki-Strickland
      Internal-External Control
      Scale), 16-17
Antonovsky, A., 4
Anxiety, 43
  in AIDS, 21-22
  cancer patients vs. physically
      healthy populations, 149
  Hospital Anxiety and Depression
      Scale (HADS), 37,38,
      142-143,147
  psychological function testing,
      129,131
  State-Trait Anxiety Inventory
      (STAI), 129-130,138-139